Mid-Life: Developmental and Clinical Issues

Mid-Life:

Developmental and Clinical Issues

Edited by

William H. Norman, Ph. D.

and

Thomas J. Scaramella, M. D.

BRUNNER/MAZEL, *Publishers* • New York

Library of Congress Cataloging in Publication Data

Main entry under title:

Mid-life, developmental and clinical issues.

  Includes bibliographies and indexes.
  1. Middle-age—Psychological aspects—Congresses.   2. Psychiatry—Congresses.
I. Norman, William H., 1946-   II. Scaramella, Thomas J., 1943-
RC451.4.M54M5   616.89   79-24367
ISBN 0-87630-221-5

Published by
BRUNNER/MAZEL, INC.
19 Union Square
New York, New York 10003

MANUFACTURED IN THE UNITED STATES OF AMERICA

Contents

Preface

This book is a direct outgrowth of a Symposium on Mid-Life that we conceived and chaired in the Spring of 1978 at Butler Hospital. Prominent academician/researchers and clinicians were invited to address the developmental and clinical implications of middle-aged adulthood with regard to their particular areas of interest. The audience responded positively to the symposium, and both professionals and lay persons were eager to learn more about the challenges, options and clinical implications of middle-aged adulthood. Each participant was invited to write a chapter based on the formal papers delivered at the symposium. The results of their efforts have been gathered and prepared specifically for this volume.

Overview of Book

Like other periods in the life cycle, the middle years of adulthood may be interpreted in various ways. Until recently, pejorative comments about the proverbial middle-age spread and the seven-year itch, as well as the emphasis among professionals on the deprivation and losses associated with aging in our culture, have predominated over more serious interest in the developmental challenges and options during the middle years of the life span. Contrary to these stereotypes, as well as to other misconceptions of adulthood, we have come to realize in the past few decades that the middle years of adulthood constitute a complex and dynamic period within the life span.

The contributors to this volume demonstrate that middle-aged adulthood encompasses more than specific years, biological changes or orchestrations of earlier adaptations. Rather, professionals are now viewing the middle years as a period in the life cycle, like other periods, in which a person's past endowments and deficits, as well as present opportunities and restraints, all interact, with consequences that influence changes in self-perception and the boundary between self and the interpersonal world.

With these ideas in mind, the book is intended to serve two major purposes. The first purpose is to provide the reader with a survey of the accumulating literature on the social and personal factors that influence not only the alterations in the rhythm and timing of life events, thus affecting perceptions of self and adaptational patterns, but also the developing personality and future life prospects.

The second purpose of this book is to alert the reader to those developmental challenges, options and potential problematic areas that have important implications in the clinical setting. It is our impression that many clinicians, while possessing some familiarity with developmental challenges of the middle years and with mid-life dynamics, often focus only on the crisis aspects of the middle years while neglecting many of the options that are also associated with mid-life—options that arise from a continually changing self and new adaptations which allow for greater individuation and self-fulfillment.

Obviously, these challenges and options do not operate equally for everyone at a given time, nor in the same degree at all times for a given individual. However, by acknowledging that middle adulthood brings with it not only crises and challenges but also options, the clinician is in a better position to assess: 1) age-related roles and age expectations that are central to the person's sense of self; 2) the extent to which the person's behavior and symptomatology are age-related or represent a deviation from earlier adaptations and unresolved conflicts; 3) the rhythm and timing of life's events that influence the person's adaptational patterns and future life prospects; and 4) the indications for therapeutic intervention.

Changes within the field of mid-life studies are occurring with such rapidity that it is impossible to speak with finality about many issues discussed in the chapters. Nevertheless, we believe that the chapters that follow bring important developmental and clinical insight to bear on the subject of adult change over time and that they provide the reader with an appraisal of the direction in which clinical advancements are being made, as well as areas in need of more rigorous investigation. It is our hope that the contributions in this volume will stimulate and enhance the reader's awareness of the complexities, challenges and options that occur during this period of the life span cycle.

Each of the nine chapters that follow examines a particular area within the field of middle adulthood development. Each chapter can be read as an up-to-date and authoritative contribution in the area it covers. Although some background in psychology and sociology is assumed, we believe that the subject matter should appeal to a wide range of students and practitioners, including psychiatrists, psychiatric residents, medical students, psychologists, social workers, mental health workers, and interested lay persons.

In Chapter 1, Nancy Datan places in historical perspective an overview of common developmental dilemmas and challenges of adulthood, as conveyed through the medium of common myths, folk and fairy tales. The author examines the developmental issues of autonomy, intimacy, achievement, and generativity and underscores their ubiquity and antiquity.

The second chapter, by Theodore Lidz, provides a general overview of the adult phases of life, including a review of important developmental tasks and critical transition periods, from the young adult phase through advanced old age. In addition, Dr. Lidz examines various developmental fixations that impair passage through the stages of adult life.

David Gutmann, in Chapter 3, takes a cross-cultural view of the post-parental years and examines the developmental potentials of middle and later life. The relevance of his data to the clinical setting is discussed. Readers interested in this area of mid-life development will find the material in this chapter helpful in their diagnostic and treatment formulations of men and women in mid-life transition.

The next chapter, by Stanley H. Cath, provides an important analysis of mid-life transitions and the suicidal person and examines in detail the prestructural determinants and potential precursors that threaten intrapsychic stability and self-cohesiveness, leading to self-annihilation. In addition, the perplexing dilemma of when threats to narcissistic vulnerability and self-cohesiveness provide barriers against self-annihilation is addressed, as well as the implications for assessment and therapeutic intervention with the suicidal person.

In Chapter 5, Malcolm B. Bowers, Jr., John Steidl, Deborah Rabinovitch, Jean W. Brenner and J. Craig Nelson examine the psychological processes which underlie the form and content of the psychotic experience, as well as the developmental challenges and stressful life circumstances surrounding the onset of the psychosis.

Malkah Notman, in Chapter 6, provides an excellent survey of the changing roles for women at mid-life and examines important developmental/adaptational pattern differences between men and women in mid-life.

Chapter 7, by Robert E. Gould, is concerned with the psychosexual developmental challenges of middle-aged adults. The chapter includes an interesting analysis of traditional sex roles and their relation to the psychosexual challenges of our current mid-life generation, who find themselves aging in a youth-obsessed culture in which mutuality and equality are valued in interpersonal relationships. Of particular clinical relevance is the discussion of sex-role conflicts and the implications for future sex-role prospects.

Chapter 8, by Carola H. Mann, concerns the strains and challenges of the middle-aged couple and the family and examines the developmental implications of these changes for the couple and their family. In addition, the chapter reviews psychodynamic theories of adult development and evaluates their applicability to marital and family issues that occur during the middle years.

Nathan W. Turner, in Chapter 9, presents an overview of the critical challenges associated with marital disenchantment during the middle years of development and examines in detail the disenchantment process, commencing with estrangement and concluding with post-divorce adjustments. A comprehensive model of separation and divorce counseling, as well as the clinical implications of this model for assessment and potential treatment applications derived from the model, are discussed. Clinicians involved in marital and divorce counseling will find this chapter particularly relevant.

ACKNOWLEDGMENTS

As with any undertaking of this sort, numerous people have assisted in bringing our initial idea to fruition. We would like to acknowledge our debt and our appreciation to Frank Delmonico, Executive Director of Butler Hospital, and Robert Westlake, M.D., acting section chairman of Psychiatry and Human Behavior, who provided the leadership and resources which allowed us to convene the symposium. We are especially indebted to Mary Moran, former Director of Public Relations, and her staff, as well as the Butler Hospital Grand Rounds Committee, whose efforts and resources contributed to the success of the symposium.

We should like to thank Tatiana Bauer, Debra Robinson, Erika Schmidt and Kathy Mechnig, for their invaluable assistance in the production of the book, and to Belinda Johnson, for reviewing parts of the manuscripts and offering her assistance.

We are especially grateful to the nine contributing authors for their patience and sustained cooperation. Finally, we express our appreciation to all those clinicians and scholars whose writings and research have inspired a new interest in mid-life development and have provided a foundation for others to build upon.

WILLIAM H. NORMAN, Ph.D.
THOMAS J. SCARAMELLA, M.D.

Contributors

MALCOLM B. BOWERS, JR., M.D.

Dr. Bowers received his B.A. degree in 1954 from Southern Methodist University and his M.D. (1958) from Washington University School of Medicine. He completed his medical internship at Fitzsimons General Hospital, Denver, in 1959 and his psychiatric residency at Yale University School of Medicine in 1965. Dr. Bowers is currently Professor of Psychiatry at Yale University School of Medicine and Chief of Psychiatry at Yale-New Haven Hospital. His primary clinical and academic interests are the experiential aspects of altered behavioral states, psychopharmacology, neurochemistry, and psychosis.

JEAN W. BRENNER, M.S.W.

Ms. Brenner received her B.A. degree from Connecticut College, her M.A. from Columbia University and her M.S.W. from the Smith College School of Social Work. She is currently Assistant Clinical Professor of Social Work in Psychiatry, Yale University School of Medicine and on the staff of Yale-New Haven Hospital, Neuropsychiatric Evaluation Unit and 90-Day Treatment Unit.

STANLEY H. CATH, M.D.

Dr. Cath received his B.S. degree from Providence College in 1942 and his M.D. (1946) from Boston University School of Medicine. In 1947, Dr. Cath completed his medical internship at Memorial

Hospital, Rhode Island. He did his psychiatric residency training in 1952 at State Hospital, Norristown, Pennsylvania, and graduated from the Boston Psychoanalytic Institute in 1958. Dr. Cath is currently Associate Clinical Professor of Psychiatry at Tufts University School of Medicine, Lecturer on Psychiatry at Boston School of Medicine and Faculty Member of the Boston Psychoanalytic Society and Institute. He is founder and medical director of the Family Advisory Service and Treatment Center Inc., a nonprofit organization designed to deal with the problems of the adult children and grandchildren of the aged population. His primary clinical and academic interests include cultism and the young, emotional disorders and suicide in middle and later years of life.

NANCY DATAN, PH.D.

Dr. Datan received her B.S. degree from Shimer College in 1959, a Masters degree (1961) and a Ph.D. (1971) degree in human development from the University of Chicago. She is currently an Associate Professor of Psychology at West Virginia University. Dr. Datan's primary interests include dynamic and social perspectives on adulthood and aging, personality changes in adulthood which accompany changes in family cycles, and conflict and transition in the life cycle of women.

ROBERT E. GOULD, M.D.

Dr. Gould received his B.A. degree from the University of Maryland in 1945 and his M.D. (1949) from the University of Virginia School of Medicine. He completed his residency at Bellevue Psychiatric Hospital in 1954 and graduated from the William Alanson White Psychoanalytic Institute in 1960. Dr. Gould is currently Associate Director of the Family Life Division of Obstetrics and Gynecology and Professor of Psychiatry at the New York Medical College. His primary clinical and academic interests are human sexuality, management of adolescent and family problems, and the changing sociocultural roles of men and women and the consequent influence on the individual, marriage, family and society.

DAVID L. GUTMANN, Ph.D.

Dr. Gutmann received his M.A. degree (1956) and his Ph.D. (1958) from the University of Chicago. He did his clinical psychology internship at the Neuro-Psychiatric Institute, University of Illinois Medical School, completing that training in 1957. He is currently Chief, Division of Psychotherapy, Northwestern University School of Medicine, Chicago, and Director of Research and Clinical Practice in the Mental Health of Later Life, Joint NUMS-University of Chicago Training Program. His primary interests involve cross-cultural research on the latter half of the human life cycle, and developmental issues in the psychological disorders of the later years.

THEODORE LIDZ, M.D.

Dr. Lidz received his A.B. degree in 1931 and M.D. (1936) from Columbia University. He did his internship at Yale-New Haven Hospital and his psychiatric residency at the Henry Phipps Psychiatric Clinic, John Hopkins Hospital, completing the residency in 1941. In 1956, Dr. Lidz graduated from the Baltimore and Western New England Psychoanalytic Institutes. He is the recipient of the Frieda Fromm-Reichmann Award, Salmon Lecturer Medal and William C. Menninger Award. Dr. Lidz is currently Sterling Professor of Psychiatry Emeritus, Yale University School of Medicine. His primary clinical and academic interests are family and human adaptation, schizophrenia and the family, and treatment of psychiatric disorders.

CAROLA H. MANN, Ph.D.

Dr. Mann received her B.A. degree in 1951 from Hunter College, a Masters degree (1953) from New School for Social Research, New York, and a Ph.D. degree (1957) in clinical psychology from the Graduate School of Arts and Sciences, New York University. In 1972, Dr. Mann graduated with a Certificate in Psychoanalysis from the William Alanson White Institute of Psychiatry, Psychoanalysis and Psychology. She is in private practice in New York City and Westchester and is a member of the teaching faculty, a supervisor of psychotherapy and Director of the Mid-Life Crisis Project at the William Alanson White Institute. Dr. Mann is a founding staff member of the Northern Westchester Center for Psychotherapy and is on the teaching and supervising faculty of the Institute for Contemporary Psychotherapy. Her primary interests are psychoanalysis, analytically-oriented psychotherapy, and the study of mid-life issues and patterns.

J. CRAIG NELSON, M.D.

Dr. Nelson received his A.B. degree from Stanford University in 1964 and his M.D. degree from the University of Wisconsin at Madison (1968). He is currently Assistant Professor of Psychiatry, Yale University School of Medicine, and Director of the Acute Psychiatric Treatment Unit, Yale-New Haven Hospital.

WILLIAM H. NORMAN, Ph.D.

Dr. Norman received his B.S. degree from Youngstown University in 1968 and a Ph.D. (1975) in Clinical Psychology from the Pennsylvania State University. In 1975, he completed his clinical internship at Duke University Medical Center, Durham, North Carolina. He is currently Director of Psychological Assessment Program, at Butler Hospital, Providence, Rhode Island, and Assistant Professor of Psychiatry, Department of Psychiatry and Human Behavior, Brown University in Providence. Dr. Norman's primary clinical and academic interests are the assessment and treatment of depression from a social learning perspective, and the development of an attribution theory model of learned helplessness.

MALKAH TOLPIN NOTMAN, M.D.

Dr. Notman received her B.S. degree from the University of Chicago in 1947 and her M.D. (1952) from Boston University School of Medicine. She did her internship at New England Center Hospital and psychiatric residency at Boston State Hospital at the Beth Israel Hospital, completing the residency in 1955. Dr. Notman graduated from the Boston Psychoanalytic Institute in 1963 and is currently Associate Clinical Professor of Psychiatry, Harvard Medical School, Staff Liaison Psychiatrist with Obstetrics and Gynecology, Beth Israel Hospital, a faculty member and Training and Supervising Analyst at the Boston Psychoanalytic Institute. Her primary clinical and academic interests are psychotherapy and women, psychoanalytic therapy in relation to women, menopause and mid-life years, psychodynamic issues for the rape victim, and psychology of pregnancy.

DEBORAH RABINOVITCH, M.S.W.

Ms. Rabinovitch received her B.A. degree from New York University in 1968 and her M.S.W. from the University of Denver Graduate School of Social Work (1973). She is currently a clinical social worker at Yale-New Haven Hospital.

THOMAS J. SCARAMELLA, M.D.

Dr. Scaramella received his A.B. from Brown University in 1965 and his M.D. (1969) from the University of Pennsylvania School of Medicine. In 1970, Dr. Scaramella completed his medical internship at Greenwich Hospital, Greenwich, Connecticut. He did his psychiatric residency training at the University of Pennsylvania Medical School, completing the residency in 1972. Dr. Scaramella is currently coordinator of psychiatry and behavioral science, Pawtucket Memorial Hospital, and Clinical Assistant Professor of Psychiatry, Department of Psychiatry and Human Behavior, Brown University. His primary clinical and academic interests are the training of physicians in psychological medicine and psychotherapy of adults and families.

JOHN STEIDL, M.S.W.

Mr. Steidel received his A.B. degree from Union College (1955), and B.D. degree from Yale University (1959), and a M.S.W. degree from Smith College School for Social Work (1971). He is currently Chief, Psychiatric Social Services, and Director of Family Therapy, Yale-New Haven Hospital, Associate Clinical Professor of Psychiatry, Yale Medical School, and Assistant Director, Dana Psychiatric Clinic.

NATHAN W. TURNER, Ed.D.

Dr. Turner received his B.A. degree (1953) from the University of Redlands, California, a Masters degree (1970) and a Ed.D. (1976) degree from Temple University. Dr. Turner completed his internship in 1973 at the Marriage Council of Philadelphia, University of Pennsylvania. He is currently an Assistant Professor of Psychiatry and Human Behavior, Jefferson Medical College, and Adjunct Professor of Ministry of Counseling, Eastern Baptist Theological Seminary. His primary clinical and academic interests are assessment and intervention with couples and treatment of marital discord.

*Mid-Life: Developmental and
Clinical Issues*

Chapter 1

Midas and Other Mid-Life Crises

Nancy Datan

Mid-life crises are in fashion today: We all know someone who is having one, or treating one, or writing a paper on the subject. Analyses of the mid-life crisis are nearly as numerous as cases of crisis, but, despite a diversity of theories, certain common themes emerge (Brim, 1974; Gould, 1978; Levinson, Darrow, Klien, Levinson and McKee, 1978). Like other transitions in the life cycle, the mid-life crisis is a product of multiple determinants. It has been traced to factors such as possible stagnation in marriage and career, declining opportunities with advancing age, and biological deficits: in brief, intrinsic and extrinsic causes, maturational, social, and existential.

It is often suggested that the crisis of meaning in middle age is,

I am indebted to Bruno Bettelheim for a critical reading of an early draft of this paper. My indebtedness extends beyond his helpful suggestions for this paper, reaching back to the inspiration I felt in 1972, when he described his own enchantment with fairy tales.

at least in part, a consequence of recent social changes and concomitant changes in the life cycle, such as increased longevity, fewer children born closer together, leaving the family nest sooner and consequently leaving the middle-aged parents with nothing to do. Children no longer fill the home and the daily routine, while affluence has removed the taste of struggle from life and simultaneously increased the availability and visibility of options, leading not only to freedom of choice but also to discontent.

These views of middle age sound like a Schoolroom Theory of Mid-Life Crisis. Teachers know that if a roomful of children are left to their own devices, they will soon be making trouble. Life span developmental theory seems to suggest that the same is true of middle-aged adults: Left to themselves, they will soon find trouble. Their maturity is demonstrated by the relocation of trouble from the interpersonal to the intrapsychic. In the rooms where the middle-aged live, quarrels are not between people but deep within the self, and the aggression of youth is turned inward, to become the depression of middle age.

I am prepared to accept the pessimistic view of human nature suggested by developmental psychology, but I am unwilling to agree that the problems of middle age are new. A dynamic perspective on the life cycle, I believe, permits us to anticipate trouble, because the dynamic perspective suggests the ubiquity of conflict, and the brevity of resolution. An abundance of clichés testifies to the conflict in the life cycle: "We get too soon old and too late smart"; "Little children, little problems—big children, big problems"; and the ultimate threat—"Wait until you grow up and have children of your own." Gould (1978) suggests that the discovery of truth in cultural clichés is one of the tasks of middle adulthood. It is my purpose to demonstrate that this discovery reaches back into antiquity, and to suggest that a recognition of the truth in cultural clichés is more than trivially interesting.

The themes of our Western myths of knowledge contain recognition of conscious self-determination, responsibility for the self and an attendant sense of loneliness, the uneasy appetite for knowledge, recognition of the necessity of work, desire for the fruits of one's own labor, and, finally, ambivalence about one's relationship to the next generation. I shall suggest that the prominent themes of our cultural heritage are also the prominent themes of the developmental transition to adulthood—from dependency to autonomy, and finally to responsibility for others—and thus, of the developmental dynamics of middle age. Although the behavioral components of this transition—commitment to career, to marriage, to children—will be addressed in subsequent chapters of the book, the purpose of this chapter is to underscore the antiquity of these issues.

I shall demonstrate the antiquity of crisis through an application of the dynamic perspective to myth, folklore, and fairy tales. A series of surprises initiated my inquiries, and, since I believe that the distinction between investigator and investigation is by no means as sharp as we like to suppose, I shall share my surprises—all the better to share my theories.

Several years ago, I was preparing a lecture on Freud's paper, "The Development of the Libido," in which his model of the Oedipus complex is derived from a sensitive analysis of Sophocles' tragedy of *Oedipus Rex* (1966). All psychologists and psychiatrists are familiar with Oedipal dynamics—the small boy who desires his mother to the exclusion of his father. I would venture to say, however, that not many have gone from Freud's lectures back to Sophocles' original drama, or they would have been as startled as I was to realize that Oedipus Rex is a play for and about adults. Sexual passion and murderous rage abound, but it is adults who are moved by these forces, beginning with the father of Oedipus, who is the only person in this tragedy to attempt premeditated murder.

King Laius, hearing the prophecy that he will be killed by his son, instructed a shepherd to take the baby out to the mountains to die. This attempted murder failed not through any weakening of the father's murderous intention, but because the shepherd was moved by compassion to save the baby, and gave him into the hands of a neighboring king. In Greek tragedy, as in dynamic psychology, one cannot escape one's doom, and so Oedipus, fleeing his foster parents' home to avert the prophecy of patricide and incest, met a stranger at the place where three roads intersect, murdered him and married his widow, and so, of course, fulfilled the prophecy in seeking to escape it.

Reading the drama with dynamic psychology in mind, I judged that we have been looking too long at little boys, and too little at their fathers and mothers. I saw the Oedipus complex as only one-half of a dynamic interaction between child and parents, in which the second half, the sexual and aggressive passions of the parents, seemed curiously neglected. For example, Erikson asserted in 1970 that "parricide remains a much more plausible explanation of the world's ills than does filicide"—a highly improbable statement in light of current statistics on child abuse, which make it all too easy to establish the ubiquity of rage and lust among adults (Justice and Justice, 1976).

Just as I had taken my first steps toward formulating a model of ongoing conflict between parent and child, it was my privilege to hear Bruno Bettelheim lecture on "The Hidden Message of the Fairy Tale" (in Jerusalem, 1972), later to become part of his book, *The Uses of Enchantment* (1976). I was captivated by his analyses, which demonstrated the ego-appropriate solutions to the dynamic dilemmas of childhood, conveyed through the medium of the fairy tale. I felt it was possible to study adult developmental dynamics as well, through attention to the adults who inhabit fairy tales—the neglected villains as well as the occasional good fairies.

In this chapter, I shall explore two dimensions of development which may find expression in mid-life crises: the individual's course of development, and the development seen in the family life cycle. I shall argue that the components of the mid-life crisis are not new: On the contrary, I will suggest that myths, folk and fairy tales carry abundant warnings about the dynamics of middle life, and describe the developmental dilemmas of adulthood in the twentieth century with an accuracy which might be called embarrassing—or eternal.

I. INDIVIDUAL DEVELOPMENT: FORBIDDEN FRUITS AND SORROW

"The love of learning is a dangerous thing, and whoever increases knowledge increases sorrow," Ecclesiastes warns the generations to come, anticipating the ambivalence which accompanies each new stage of growth and development in the individual life cycle, with its mixed blessings of autonomy, mastery, and power—and the attendant loss of dependency. The testimony for this claim is written across human history, from prehistoric myths to contemporary accounts of riots on university campuses.

I believe that the story of the Garden of Eden and the record of student riots share significant elements, reflecting aspects of a major transition in adult personality development: the transition from dependency to an awareness of self-determination and reliance upon the self. Two aspects of this transition can be seen in the ancient story of the Garden of Eden and the recent history of student riots: an irresistible desire for knowledge, and pain as the price of this knowledge—the price of self-consciousness and responsibility. These are two major components of the dialectical dynamics of the transition into adulthood.

I propose that this transition into adulthood is best seen in the context of a developmental model of personality. I see this transition as a passage from dependency to responsibility, and from innocence to knowledge. This passage can be seen on three dimensions: in the transition to self-sufficiency represented by the story of the Garden of Eden; in the search for mastery over nature represented by the story of Prometheus; and in the price of power, represented by the legend of Midas and the tale of the Fisherman's Wife.

While the self and its solitude are major themes in existential psychology, the developmental model of the transition to adulthood has focused on the fit between self and society. Erikson's discussions of identity and youth (1963; 1964; 1965; 1970) deal with commitment to or alienation from society, and this is the perspective taken by subsequent writers such as Keniston (1970). The problem of young adulthood, in developmental theory, is often conceived in sociological terms. It would be unkind but not at all untrue to say that a brief overview of Erikson's (1963) description of the core problem in ego development, identity versus role confusion, might lead the reader to conclude that the problem of ego identity can be resolved by competent career counseling.

It is not my intention to deny or even to diminish the importance of fit between self and society, but I shall argue that the external process of role commitment is a manifestation of an internal process in which the individual moves from the dependency of infancy and childhood toward the independence of adolescence and young adulthood, and finally to the point of responsibility for the new and dependent generation to come. This maturationally-determined series of transformations can be discerned in the life cycle of all animal species not wholly governed by instinct, and it takes on increasing complexity as we ascend the phylogenetic scale.

"It is human to have a long childhood," Erikson remarks (1963); the uniquely prolonged childhood of human beings is mandated by our slow growth. This is the time when parents teach their children, since instincts do not; it is easy to see the evolutionary advantage of a prolonged childhood for our behaviorally plastic species. Parents may, if necessary, impose their instructions by force on the small child. This advantage is illustrated if we consider the alternative: an angry child who wants the cookie jar, and who, like the horse, has reached adult size at two years of age.

If the long dependency of childhood is shaped by biological imperatives, the child's transition to adulthood is arbitrarily determined by cultural patterns within the very broad context bounded by biology. While betrothal may occur at or before birth in some cultures, cohabitation, even in primitive societies, comes with sexual maturity. Prolonged adolescence and youth can be seen in societies such as our own, where physical maturity comes in the teens, legal adulthood is set by political decree at eighteen years, and economic and social maturity may not come until several additional years of dependency and apprenticeship have passed. This long, ambiguous transition, it is often suggested, creates ambivalence and insecurity in young adulthood.

I am not convinced that the ambiguity of transition in contemporary society engenders ambivalence in young adulthood, nor do I hold the related belief that this particular set of growing pains is part of the malaise of modernity. It is my contention that both desire and doubt concerning the independence which comes with biological maturity can be seen in our best-known myths, and that ambivalence has marked the transition to maturity since the beginning of Western culture. While twentieth-century technology facilitates expressions of doubt, and our comparative affluence and its attendant options may cause conflicts to become more salient, the crises of adult life so prominent in current developmental psychology are foreshadowed in ancient myths.

The sense of the self and its solitude as a normative developmental phenomenon is a common theme in descriptions of middle age, such as the increased interiority of personality (Neugarten et al., 1964), the personalization of death (Neugarten, 1968), and the awareness of oneself as the head of the line (Jacques, 1965). I propose that these themes first emerge in young adulthood, and that the developmental tensions between individual growth and the needs of the next generation which may create a crisis in middle life are best understood as integral components of the transition to maturity.

Adam and Eve: The Price of Maturity

I have never been comfortable with Erikson's (1963) notion that we bite into the apple of Eden with our baby teeth, and forfeit paradise before we can stand upright. My daughters fueled my doubts when they brought home their own versions of the story of Adam and Eve from their Israeli kindergarten and first grade. The Hebrew verb פתה encompasses persuasion and seduction: hence, my second-born daughter, at five, asked: "The woman persuaded/seduced her husband, right?" and added, with evident pride, "Then she was the *first* to eat"—rewriting, with one bold stroke, two thousand years' interpretation of Woman as Sinner.

Not long afterward, my firstborn daughter came home from first grade with the *chutzpah* of latency: "I want to eat from the fruit of the Tree of Knowledge." Against mythic desires, motherhood pales: I asked her, "Don't you think that's what happens when you go to school?" "But I want my eyes to be opened *all* the way."

Mothers and daughters are unrepresented in the ranks of the Talmudic scholars. I offer this narrative not as a revision of Biblical interpretation but as the context in which I first became aware of the sexual and intellectual passions in the story of the Garden of Eden. I pursued the questions my children had raised by asking my students in developmental psychology to tell me the story of the Garden of Eden. Over the years, not one student has been unable to tell me the story—but not one has told it accurately yet. The story my students tell is this: There was a tree in the center of the Garden of Eden whose fruit gave knowledge of good and evil. This tree was forbidden to Adam and Eve, but the serpent tempted Eve and she took the fruit, ate of it, and persuaded Adam to eat. For their transgressions, Eve was punished with the pain of childbirth and Adam condemned to labor for his bread, and both were expelled from the Garden of Eden.

This retelling includes every element of the tale but one, and I think the omission is not insignificant. In all my years of teaching, I have not yet heard a student spontaneously recall—though all remember it when reminded—that Adam and Eve were expelled from the Garden of Eden so as to prevent their obtaining the fruit of the second forbidden tree, the Tree of Life. I am prepared to conclude that if we were given a second chance in the Garden of Eden—as each of us is, in every generation—we would make straight for the Tree of the Knowledge of Good and Evil once again: for knowledge, however dangerous, is evidently a more potent temptation than immortality.

I reject, therefore, Erikson's reading of this story (1963). He suggests that the oral stage of development may be the ontogenetic contribution to the story of Adam and Eve, who in biting the apple lost paradise—as does the infant, Erikson proposes, when his teeth come through. I doubt that paradise is lost so swiftly, and I suggest that the prominent theme in the story of Adam and Eve is the forced transition from dependency, where all is provided, into the wider world of love and work—the tasks of the healthy adult. Despite the centuries of technological progress since the story of Adam and Eve first found expression—centuries which have seen the mitigation of women's woe in childbirth through modern medicine, and the conquest of sweat by Madison Avenue—this tale continues to tell us about the one-way, bitter, but tempting road into adulthood.

Prometheus: The Price of Technology

Nietzsche has argued in *The Birth of Tragedy* that the story of Adam and Eve, with its dependency, seduction, and deceit, represents the feminine element in humanity. He contrasts this femininity unfavorably with the "higher" masculinity of Prometheus—an active defiance of the gods, not the passive disobedience in response to persuasion. Prometheus deceived Zeus and stole fire from the gods, bringing its light and the light of astronomy, mathematics, and early argiculture to humanity. For his sins the punishment was correspondingly more grave: not expulsion from paradise, but an eternity of torment. He was chained to a rock, his entrails devoured each day; and each night the devoured flesh grew back so that the torture could continue; his only hope lay in the prophecy that one day his chains would fall away of themselves.

Current concerns over destructive technology and its threats to our environment bear out the message of the myth of Prometheus, rather than the hopes of the mythical Prometheus himself or the judgment of Nietzsche. Indeed, the history of technology indicates that controversy almost always accompanies a major scientific advance. Resistance often takes the form of concern over damage to nature, and sooner or later, it seems, this concern is often justified.

Furthermore, the advances of civilized technology fail to deliver their promise of spiritual reward. Freud remarked in 1930 that man with all his devices had the splendor of a prosthetic god, and yet it seemed to bring him no happiness (1962). While Freud predicted continuing dramatic advances in technology, he also warned that present-day man was ill at ease with his magnificence. Almost half a century has passed since Freud issued this warning, and it would seem that humanity has come no closer to happiness, while Freud is no farther from truth.

Like Adam and Eve, however, Prometheus is impelled by irresistible forces which appear to be universal, for, like the myth of the Fall from a natural environment where all is provided, the myth of stolen knowledge is found in all civilizations (Campbell, 1970). We have no myths at all, however, in which there is a voluntary restoration of the status quo, a return of stolen knowledge in exchange for lost innocence and dependency. Nor have we heard a majority yet declare its willingness to renounce mastery over nature in exchange for the ecological balance of an earlier age. Like knowledge, mastery over nature is a theme with many variations in our mythologies, including our current developmental mythologies of middle age. Through all its variations, a common theme is found: conquest and consequences, the first irresistible, the second inevitable.

Midas and the Mid-Life Crisis of Achievement

The tale of the Garden of Eden records the most primitive of truths: the transition from dependency to toil and autonomy. The legend of Prometheus reflects a measure of progress, for the knowledge obtained by Prometheus is meant to lead to mastery over nature and a mitigation of the curse of Adam and Eve. The dynamics of the mid-life crisis are anticipated in these cultural messages which describe individual growth toward autonomy and achievement. Ambivalence about knowledge and mastery runs through these stories, and it is this ambivalence—a combination of greed and anticipated despair—which is captured by the myth of Midas, a myth about wealth and its consequences.

In Midas we see a man who has gone beyond the struggle for subsistence to accumulate an effortless surplus. Midas was born of a union between a nameless satyr—the species which gave its name to the state of surplus sexual passion—and the Great Goddess of Ida. While he was still an infant in the cradle, an omen foretold a future of wealth. The prophecy was fulfilled when Midas grew into adulthood: He extended hospitality to the debauched satyr Silenus, and thus found favor with Dionysus, whom the Greeks credit with discovering wine and divine madness. Dionysus asked Midas how he would like to be rewarded, and Midas requested that all he touch turn to gold. His wish was granted, and before long, he had touched his lunch and deprived himself of the sustenance of food, and touched his beloved daughter and deprived himself of the sustenance of love. Like so many other folk heroes, Midas begged to be released from his wish; Dionysus, much amused, granted his request.

Midas, in going beyond subsistence, achieved wealth—and with it complete impoverishment, a perversion of excess. And yet the excess of Midas was simply an excess of mastery, a complete instead of a partial victory in the struggle to win subsistence. Nevertheless, the parallels between Midas and those whom we describe today as workaholics, whose dedication to work and its rewards at the expense of the inner self and its needs, are sufficiently close to persuade me that the mid-life crisis of affluence and achievement is not new. Current developmental and clinical portraits of the impoverished inner self in middle life (Gould, 1978) are foreshadowed in the myth of Midas and others like him, who carry their wishes just a little too far, and come to grief—a grief as old as human legends, and not a product of our times.

The Fisherman's Wife

King Midas knew when to stop, but other folk tales record the fate of men and women who did not. Of these, one is the fisherman's wife, who was able to move from her hovel of poverty, through the powers of a magical fish her husband had caught and mercifully returned to the sea. But her cottage gave her no pleasure; she sent her husband back to the seashore to ask for a palace. Next she asked to be emperor, then Pope, and finally she told her husband to command the fish to make her God. With this last wish the skies clouded over, and the fisherman's wife found herself once again in her poor hovel by the sea.

If the greed of Midas is the forerunner of the empty inner life of the middle-aged workaholic, then the poverty of the fisherman's wife, whose demands on her husband have no bounds, is a forewarning to the housewives of the suburbs, who sometimes discover their palaces to be empty, impoverished shells. Jessie Bernard's provocative comments on the future of marriage (1973) suggest that the bargain struck in the traditional marriage is less than equitable: The enhanced psychological well-being of the married man, when compared to the single man, is achieved at the expense of the mental health of the married woman, who is disadvantaged compared to the single woman. This bargain, which is under critical scrutiny by contemporary feminists, suggests that a woman surrenders independence for comfort and protection. The message of the tale of the fisherman's wife, as well as of contemporary family sociology, is that this exchange may carry its own seeds of doom.

While the flaws in women's myths of dependency and security are becoming evident, the complementary myths of men are not yet being explored. The woman who hopes to find complete happiness in a comfortable home is matched by the man whose workday is spent in the belief that he provides it.* The fisherman, sent to the seashore again and again by his wife's insatiable dreams of power, is fortunate to discover himself a victim of nothing worse than his original poverty, when his drama of marital greed has been played out. The fate of contemporary partners in similar dramas can be less kind. Young executives on the rise, suddenly dead of early heart attacks or other stress-related illnesses, testify to the unexamined price paid by men in a marital exchange which brings losses to both partners. As other contributors to this volume will show, these ancient expectations are undergoing changes which will benefit both women and men.

II. THE FAMILY AT MID-LIFE: A BIRD-WATCHER'S GUIDE TO THE EMPTY NEST

Conventional wisdom in developmental psychology suggests that the trials of the earlier stages in the family life cycle culminate in the tribulations of the empty nest. This choice of idiom invites our critical scrutiny: Birdwatchers know that fledglings are pushed from the nest by their parents. Myth, folk, and fairy tales, from Oedipus Rex to Snow White, provide familiar cultural idioms suggesting that human parents may do the same, a suggestion which finds support in anthropological observations of infanticide (Harris, 1977), as well as the growing problem of child abuse in this country (Bakan, 1971). The dark side of parental passions, no secret to police and social workers, is insufficiently appreciated in developmental psychology; and it is to this dimension of the parent-child relationship that I wish to turn, looking for lessons about adult developmental needs in myth and fairy tales.

Merciless Parents

A child enters the world at the mercy of its parents—a phrase underscored if we remember one of history's most merciless and misunderstood fathers, the celebrated father of the inadvertent pat-

---

* I owe thanks to Dean Rodeheaver, who has taught me that men's myths are no less consequential—though unfortunately less often explored—than the myths of women.

ricide, Oedipus Rex. It is a curious commentary on our personal mythologies that, with a little initial squeamishness, we have absorbed Oedipal murder into the developmental sequence of childhood while censoring Laius out of our image of fatherhood. It might be argued that in the drama itself Oedipus' accidental murder of his father despite his efforts to escape the dreadful prophecy overshadows Laius' deliberate plan to murder his infant son. But no such defense can be offered for Medea, whose murder of her children is the climax of a play of which she is the central figure—the heroine, according to audiences who, we might surmise, have been agreeing for 2500 years that if pushed too far they would kill their children too.

The adversary relationship between parent and child expressed by these myths reflects an underlying biological conflict between individual survival and species survival. The bearing and rearing of children serve the species whether or not they serve the individual. And indeed personal desire for children is no protection against risk: Loving mothers can die in childbirth too. If biological reproduction is accompanied by a measure of personal danger, it is hardly surprising to find this conflict manifest at the intrapsychic level as well, where the needs of the adult may clash with the needs of the offspring.

Empty Cupboards

The story of Hansel and Gretel is an example of the conflict between parents and children as it might find expression early in the family life cycle. Bettelheim (1976) sees this as a tale of children who regress to primitive oral needs, seeking limitless satiation in the gingerbread house in the woods—which proves to be inhabited by a wicked witch. They overcome her and their own infantile needs, and are then able to return home triumphant.

I find the parents' motives of interest. Hansel and Gretel are sent out of their home and into the woods by their father and stepmother because there is not enough food at home—a scarcity not confined to fairy tales or to the pantry. Faced with the boundless neediness of the very young child, what parent has not sometimes feared a scarcity—whether of money, time, energy, or in the cupboards of the heart? The ubiquity of this fear finds expression in a curious social readiness to condemn couples who elect to remain childless. Such couples are often condemned as "selfish," and the cure—curiouser and curiouser—is seen as having children. This hazardous treatment is a kind of folk testimony that children take and take, and thus deplete reserves, whether or not they successfully cure adult selfishness. And yet the childless couple is guilty of nothing more serious than accuracy at arithmetic; any finite quantity, divided by two, yields more than when it is divided by three—and the demands of children may expose the parents' resources as inadequate.

Grown Children

Dependency diminishes as childhood ends; but conflict, rather than ceasing, takes a new form. My own moment of personal discovery came when my firstborn daughter reached adolescence and the family went, as we had so often done before, to see Walt Disney's *Snow White*. Some may be surprised, and others share my surprise, to discover that my sympathies had suddenly transferred themselves to the witch.

Where the small child threatens finite resources, the maturing child threatens to take over. And indeed, in time, the normative course of the individual life cycle ends in death, with surviving children; the parent bereaved of children is a tragic figure. Nevertheless, the orderly succession of generations is not necessarily seen by the older generation as a happy ending. The adolescent, we might surmise, threatens the parent on a more primitive level than does the small infant, for the infant's needs require an omnipotent parent, while the adolescent's vigor threatens to underscore the parent's finitude and mortality. Faced by her own vanishing youth in the person of her blossoming stepdaughter, Snow White's stepmother acts on the ambivalent rage that may stir in many mothers, and finally succeeds in halting her daughter's transition to adulthood with the long sleep of the poisoned apple.

Bettelheim (1976), sees Snow White as the expression of the Oedipal conflicts which revive in adolescence, and must be mastered for the transition into sexual maurity and adulthood: Snow White is wakened by a kiss into a happy ending. It is not only the child, however, who must renounce the magic Oedipal ties to the parent; the parent too must renounce the child. And the child's renunciation is facilitated by the presence of alternate objects of love. The parent's renunciation, by contrast, is not facilitated but is mandated by the fact that the small child, once loved so tenderly and so completely, is no longer there. The small child's place has been taken by a large, vigorous youth—a possible object of sexual desire, as incest taboos and incidents testify, but no longer a possible object of parental tenderness and nurturant care, and slipping swiftly out of the reach of parental control. This period, when the children are grown but not yet out of the home, might well be called the period of the *crowded nest*—a period fully as interesting as the widely studied period of the empty nest.

Regret over departing children is not a theme in our folk inheritance. Indeed, quite the opposite is true: Children of all ages are turned out of the home. They are too hungry, too beautiful, too dangerous; if they threaten parental resources, they are sent away or killed. If the hidden message of the fairy tale for the listening child is that soon he must make his own way in the world (Bettelheim, 1976), the message adults have been sharing is no less clear: Parenthood ends when the children are grown. The period of the empty nest, interpreted by demographers of the family (Glick, 1955) as a consequence of recent changes in family spacing and concomitant changes in longevity—children born sooner and departing earlier, parents surviving longer—can thus be seen to have developmental meaning as well, which reaches further back into human history. Like the mid-life crisis of achievement, the empty nest of middle life is not a phenomenon of modernity but a theme echoing through Western culture for centuries.

III. CONCLUSION: BEYOND THE TWENTIETH CENTURY

I have suggested that of the multiple determinants of the mid-life crisis, many are not new. A brief overview of our common myths, folk and fairy tales has suggested developmental themes in the struggle for autonomy, intimacy, achievement, and generativity which are entirely consonant with current clinical and developmental models of the mid-life crisis. It is my belief that a life-span developmental psychology exclusive of historical and social change is sterile; at the same time, a developmental model dependent largely on historical and social change is transient. It has been my concern to trace the origins of certain common developmental themes in the mid-life crisis, and to suggest that our cultural heritage is fully as rich with insights as our current psychologies of middle age.

It is certainly true that the study of contemporary social change can contribute to an understanding of crisis in middle age. Consider, for example, a woman now in her 40s who chose 20 years ago to give up her career for the sake of her husband and children. She currently faces the statistical possibility of divorce and the developmental certainty of departing children—and with these two primary roles gone, a climate of opinion which is likely to add insult to injury with the suggestion that it was all a mistake in the first place to sacrifice anything for personal development. Our understanding of such an individual is surely enhanced by a knowledge of recent social changes, which have rendered once-reasonable decisions now obsolete, At the same time, I would argue that it is equally essential to recognize that the conflict between the personal needs of a woman and the contextual needs of marriage and children is at least as old as the legend of Medea.

Similarly, the executive at the peak of his career who faces a sudden crisis of meaning is surely a part of the context of the contemporary affluence, along with the "one-life, one-career imperative" (Sarason, 1977). Nevertheless, our understanding of his dilemma is incomplete without an awareness of its ubiquity and antiquity: A coupling of knowledge and doom, of power and doom, of wealth and doom, of greed and doom, is as old as Adam, as old as Prometheus, as old as Midas, as old as the Fisherman's Wife. A recognition of the developmental context of the crises of middle age must begin with an acknowledgment of ancient case histories.

REFERENCES

AESCHYLUS: *Prometheus Bound.*
BAKAN, D.: *Slaughter of the Innocents.* San Francisco: Jossey-Bass, 1971.
BERNARD, J.: *The Future of Marriage.* New York: World (Bantam), 1973.
BETTELHEIM, B.: *The Uses of Enchantment.* New York: Alfred A. Knopf, 1976.

BRIM, O. G.: Selected theories of the male mid-life crisis: A comparative overview. Invited address to Division 20, American Psychological Association, New Orleans, September 1974.

CAMPBELL, J.: The Masks of God: Primitive Mythology. New York: Viking, 1970.

ECCLESIASTES 1:18; 9:16.

ERIKSON, E. H.: Childhood and Society, (2nd ed.). New York: W. W. Norton, 1963.

ERIKSON, E. H.: Insight and Responsibility. New York: W. W. Norton, 1964.

ERIKSON, E. H.: Youth: Fidelity and diversity. In E. H. Erikson (Ed.), The Challenge of Youth. New York: Anchor Books, 1965.

ERIKSON, E. H.: Reflections on the dissent of contemporary youth. International Journal of Psychoanalysis, 1970, 51, 11-22.

EURIPIDES: Medea.

FREUD, S.: Civilization and Its Discontents. New York: W. W. Norton, 1962.

FREUD, S.: Lecture xxi: The development of the libido and the sexual organizations. The Complete Introductory Lectures on Psychoanalysis. New York: W. W. Norton, 1966.

GENESIS 2:8-3:24.

GLICK, P. C.: Life cycle of the family. Marriage and Family Relations, 1955, 17:3-9.

GOULD, R.: Transformations: Growth and Change in Adult Life. New York: Simon & Schuster, 1978.

HARRIS, M.: Cannibals and Kings. New York: Random House, 1977.

JACQUES, E.: Death and the mid-life crisis. International Journal of Psychoanalysis, 1965, 46:502-514.

JUSTICE, B. & JUSTICE, R.: The Abusing Family. New York: Human Sciences Press, 1976.

KENISTON, K.: Youth as a stage of life. American Scholar, 1970, 39:631-654.

LEVINSON, D. J., with DARROW, C. N., KLEIN, E. B., LEVINSON, M. H., & McKEE, B.: The Seasons of a Man's Life. New York: Alfred A. Knopf, 1978.

NEUGARTEN, B. L. & ASSOCIATES: Personality in Middle and Late Life. New York: Atherton Press, 1964.

NEUGARTEN, B. L.: The awareness of middle age. In B. L. Neugarten (Ed.), Middle Age and Aging. Chicago: University of Chicago Press, 1968.

NIETZSCHE, F. W.: The Birth of Tragedy. (trans. F. Golfing). New York: Doubleday, 1956.

SARASON, S. B.: Work, Aging, and Social Change: Professionals and the One Life-One Career Imperative. New York: The Free Press, 1977.

SOPHOCLES: Oedipus Rex.

Chapter 2

Phases of Adult Life: An Overview

Theodore Lidz

There is an increasing awareness that personality development does not stop with the completion of adolescence, and even less with the attainment of so-called "genital sexuality." We now appreciate that persons continue to be faced with new developmental challenges throughout the life span, new critical tasks that must be surmounted as they move from one phase to the next, and that they may undergo a profound reorientation in their attitudes toward life and themselves as they enter each new phase of life.

The passage through the various stages of adult life rests upon the manner in which persons mastered the phases of childhood and adolescence. In the study of child and adolescent development, the epigenetic principle is extremely important, for the ability to cope with the critical tasks of any phase depends on the reasonable mastery of the preceding stage. The process is essentially one of progressive separation and individuation: the gradual internalizing of directives, knowledge, and skills to gain increasing structure, integration and capacity for self-guidance. However, there are also panphasic influences—the intrafamilial, the socioeconomic and the cultural environments in which the child grows up are major determinants of the developing personality.

To state matters briefly, I might say almost symbolically, a person at the start of adult life should have attained an ego identity (Erikson, 1950) which is a summation and integration of all of his or her previous identifications and identities, and which provides a consistency that characterizes an individual despite changes that occur over time and despite the many different roles assumed at any one period in life. Young adults should also have achieved a capacity for intimacy; their experiences within their families will have fostered sufficient independence and adequately firm self-boundaries that they need not fear, but rather seek interdependence with another. It is also important for them to have overcome the cognitive egocentricity of childhood to realize that other persons feel and perceive differently than they or members of their family do. It is also important to overcome the egocentricity characteristic of adolescence to realize that solving problems subjectively, even if carefully planned and thought through, is a very different matter from solving them in actuality, and to recognize that it is necessary to move into action to gain one's goals whether in love or in a career.

It is customary to divide adult life into a young adult period, middle age, and old age, with each period divided into various substages. The periods and substages are not as set as those of childhood and adolescence and the epigenetic principle is not as pertinent. Students of adult life may divide adulthood somewhat differently but there is reasonable agreement concerning the nature of the crucial tasks that confront persons and the critical transitions in their outlook that are apt to occur as they move through the adult years.

THE YOUNG ADULT

The age at which adult life begins varies. Young persons sooner or later, usually early in their 20s, come to realize that the time has come to make commitments and that these commitments will determine to a very great extent how their future lives will go. They are apt to feel that all that has gone before is prelude and life now begins in earnest. Of course, some have made critical decisions earlier and have decided on what careers they will follow, as well as whom they will marry, while others caught up in the awareness of human malleability will require a moratorium (Erikson, 1956) before committing themselves. Such moratoria can sometimes extend into a more or less permanent ego diffusion with the absence of the commitments needed to make life truly meaningful. For some, however, a moratorium is essential, and it is useful to follow Keniston (1974) and insert a stage of Youth for those who, having gained an ego identity, become caught up in tensions between the self and society and may struggle throughout their 20s to overcome the disparity between their emergent selves and the social order.

A critical task of personality development during Youth lies in achieving individuation (Jung, 1965) —the ability to acknowledge reality and cope with it, either through acceptance or revolutionary opposition, but preserving an intactness of "self" distinct from society. Failure to individuate properly can lead to a denial of the self often resulting in overconformity, with the opposite danger lying in alienation in which efforts to preserve autonomy lead to withdrawal from the social matrix. The concept of a period of Youth is also helpful in understanding those young people who become caught up in problems of relativism (Lidz, 1976). Gaining perspective from the study of other cultures and other times, and recognizing the validity of the ways and beliefs of other peoples, they appreciate that the standards of their own society are more or less arbitrary. They wonder about their obligation to adhere to societal norms and, recognizing the relativity of values and meanings, find it difficult to gain purpose and direction. Further, awareness that what they or anyone becomes depends largely upon how and where they are brought up leads some to believe in their omnipotentiality—that they can make of themselves what they wish, and this apparent freedom to choose can be almost paralyzing.

The problems of contemporary female youth have been accentuated through their newly gained freedom in the choice of future roles. The ability to separate, with security, sex and procreation permits them to lead active sexual lives and also to decide when and if they will have children, which, together with the high level of education available to them, enables women to enter many careers formerly closed to them. They can decide between becoming house-wives and mothers or almost any career open to men. They have gained a considerable sense of their omnipotentiality, but they lack role models to follow into some careers, and the need to make the critical choice between career and motherhood can create con-siderable indecision and conflict.

During the early phase of young adult life, usually between the ages of 18 and 30, most consider that the time has come to make commitments which will greatly determine the course of the remain-der of their lives. Some young people will feel, perhaps in an exag-gerated way, that everything that has happened to them has largely been preparation, but now the time has come to start life in earnest. Sooner or later, though, the two critical commitments of choosing an occupation and a mate will start them on their way. Both choices will influence greatly the further development of their personalities and their chances for a happy future.

While the choice of an occupation depends greatly upon per-sonality characteristics, the occupation chosen will in turn greatly influence the further development of the personality. Occupational choice is generally one of two types. In one, the occupation is an expansion of the self as in the professions and arts, and major satis-factions come from the occupation; in the other, a person primarily seeks to make a living, support a family and gain security, whereas satisfactions and enjoyments are sought elsewhere—from the chil-dren, sports, or avocations. People's occupations greatly influence with whom they associate, the goals they pursue, the social roles they fill, and the ethical standards that become very much an integral part of them. The occupation selects out characteristics to be strengthened and provides patterns of living. An individual may have the potential to become a physicist, physician, engineer, but the sort of person he eventually becomes will differ according to which career he chooses.

As noted, the problem of occupational choice for women currently poses particular difficulties. For many women, occupational choice is a relatively secondary matter as marriage and motherhood are dominant goals, but serious conflict can ensue when a young woman attempts to decide whether to pursue a career or profession, or to marry and have children. Those who decide upon both career and motherhood may find the rewards of choosing both to be eminently fulfilling and gratifying but they must also be aware that unless they are extremely fortunate, serious difficulties and frustrations will be encountered. The potentiality does not depend upon the liberation of the specific woman alone but very much upon the choice of a husband who will share parental responsibilities and foster the wife's career.

The choice of a marital partner is not a necessary step in the life cycle and persons can lead happy and satisfactory lives without marrying, but as approximately 97 percent of people in the United States marry, relatively few mentally and physically competent persons never marry. There are many reasons why people marry. The desire to have a spouse rests upon the human's biological makeup and the need for prolonged nurturance in the family of origin. In the family in which children grow up, they can feel secure because their well-being is as important, if not more important, to their parents than the parents' welfare, and because, by and large, they are accepted simply because they are their parents' children rather than because of their achievements. The child's movement to become a separate and independent individual always has some conscious or unconscious counterweight pulling back toward dependency and a complete relatedness to another. After achieving and enjoying independence from parents, persons come to feel alone and insecure, and wish once again to have another to whom his or her well-being is all important.

In marriage, the spouses' lives are, at least theoretically, interdependent, and the well-being of each depends on the well-being of the other. Further, it is a relationship in which acceptance again depends primarily upon affection rather than on achievement. The two sexes are not only suited to each other for the satisfactory release of sexual tensions, but, at least until recently, the developmental process everywhere prepared males and females to fill complementary roles and functions. Persons have been so brought up that they feel and usually are incomplete unless interdependent with a member of the opposite sex, particularly in rearing children and providing for them. A major impulsion to marriage derives, however, from the unconscious desire to complete the oedipal strivings that had been frustrated in the family of origin and to be able to unite love and sex, and to become the husband or wife rather than a member of the childhood generation in the family. Marriage clearly starts a new phase in a person's life, a new way of living with a new status and set of responsibilities.

The union that is formed changes, or at least should change, the self-structure of both partners so that henceforth it concerns the direction and well-being of two lives rather than one, and superego directives as well as id impulsions of the spouse modify the behavior of the partner. The choice of a spouse is one of the most significant decisions made in a life. In most societies, the choice is considered too important to be made by an inexperienced person who is under the sway of passion, and elders make the decision. In our society, love is expected to be an important if not a major motivation, though clearly other factors usually enter into the selection. Indeed, it is a highly overdetermined matter and, in a sense, the result of each individual's total life experiences. The process of falling in love depends upon unconscious determinants that trail all the way back into infancy. Unconscious processes, however, may be more suited for weighing the diffuse needs and intangible memories that enter into the process than conscious deliberation, even if all of the variables were available for conscious consideration. Nevertheless, logical appraisals and the impressions and opinions of family and friends usually enter into making the decision about moving from being in love to marriage. Currently, increasing numbers of persons try living together before making the commitment to marriage.

Most marriages are followed by a period of readjustment upon which much of the success of a marriage may depend. The topic of marital adjustment is a large one and it encompasses far more than the sexual, even though the sexual adjustment of the couple is extremely important for a good sexual relationship serves as a lubricant to reduce frictions arising elsewhere and lack of sexual fulfillment is likely to aggravate other sources of conflict. Marital problems shortly after marriage as well as throughout life are apt to be major factors in emotional disorders even though much of the difficulty stems from earlier problems, or is an almost inevitable outcome of the choice of a spouse.

Various developmental fixations and shortcomings can impair the marital adjustment—anaclitic dependency, gender identity problems, unresolved oedipal attachments. The spouses should gain gratification from satisfying the other and being needed by the other, and not simply from being gratified and cared for. Nevertheless, many marriages succeed because the weaknesses of one or both partners are supported by the strengths of the other partner.

A new marriage is in many respects a fusion of the two families in which the partners grew up into a new pattern congenial to both members. The expectations of the marital partner, the roles assumed, the tacit understandings, the unconscious communications, and many other matters that are simply taken for granted in a family are often very disparate in the two families from which the spouses have emerged. The tendency to transfer problems with parents as well as assets of parents to a spouse is, of course, a common source of conflict and disappointment. The center of gravity in the lives of the spouses properly shifts from the families of origin and peer groups to the new family, though in some ethnic and socioeconomic groups the activities and roles of the men and women tend to remain quite discrete (Bott, 1955).

Parenthood is a state that greatly modifies the course of a person's life and which sooner or later is bound to create problems for one or both spouses (Benedek, 1959). It is likely to usher in a greater change in the life pattern than marriage itself. Whereas a marriage can exist in many divergent forms and allow the spouses great latitude in pursuing their lives as long as the relationship is satisfactory or acceptable to both, the birth of a child transforms the marriage into a family and places limitations on the roles and activities of the spouses if the well-being of the child is to be taken into consideration. It can also create frictions as one spouse or the other feels neglected in favor of the child and cannot really make room in the marriage for a child, or the difficulties in raising a child undermine one's self-esteem. Of course, children serve to strengthen many marriages.

Most women gain a deep sense of fulfillment from the creation of a child. Women's sexuality is more complicated than men's. They are consciously and unconsciously in close touch with procreation because of the menstrual cycle and their sexuality encompasses conception, the filled womb, childbirth, and nursing as well as the sexual act. Many women feel they would be incomplete without producing and nurturing a child. If the mother had felt deprived at not having been a boy, she now feels compensated, though some mothers who have little self-esteem because they are women can only gain a sense of completion by bearing a son. The child affords that profound gratification derived from knowing that one is necessary to another being, and from being loved for having given of oneself. The father also usually gains great gratification from becoming a parent. To some, having a child provides a sign of masculinity that is almost essential to the maintenance of self-esteem among some ethnic groups. On the other hand, it also permits the man some opportunity to express his nurturant feelings gained from his early identification with his mother, feelings which often have few acceptable outlets. The child will also provide the father with narcissistic supplies through his or her adulation of the father. Nevertheless, deep rivalries with a child for the wife's attention and affection can unleash old oedipal and sibling rivalries that interfere with paternal feelings. Children can provide a source of renewal to the marriage, a source of common identification between the spouses, for the child is a product of their common creativity and an object of their common interest and aspirations. The requirements of parenthood keep changing with the child's life cycle and require malleability in the parents to adapt to the child's changing needs and developing abilities, but the continuous change also affords a constant source of new interest.

THE MIDDLE YEARS

As young adults move into their 30s, they usually undergo a reorientation in their attitudes toward life. One can consider the start of the thirties as a transition to the middle years leading up to the onset of middle age around the age of 40. A fair proportion of individuals feel their youth has ended and more definitive commitments must be made. Some, unhappy about the choice of a career, decide that the time has come for a change. Marriages may be disturbed by what has been termed the "seven year itch." In general, however, persons are likely to enjoy a sense of mastery. They are now established in their own families, and feel really free from parental control. Having gained the necessary knowledge and skills to "settle in" at their occupations, they become concerned with "making it" (Levinson, 1977; Levinson, Darrow, Klein, Levinson, & McKee, 1978). They realize that just how far they get in their 30s will determine to a very great extent their ultimate success. They assume increasing responsibility and, though most are usually still considered junior members in their occupation, this is the time when truly creative persons show their capacities.

Women who have been making their way in their careers now recognize that if they wish to have children the time has come to have them. Difficult decisions and changes must be made. Those who have children now have gained the skills needed to bring a second or third child through infancy and early childhood without feeling overwhelmed. Some whose children are now in school will return to the careers they had interrupted to become mothers, whereas others will begin to prepare for a career for the first time—a shift that is very different from the pattern of men's lives at this stage of life. Women's life patterns during these years are so variant that generalizations are difficult to make.

As persons, particularly men with careers, move past the age of 35, the ambitious become impatient at being subordinates and they are apt to enter a phase in which they are impatient to "become one's own man." They may enter upon a period of intense striving to gain a promotion. Some will grow resentful, and perhaps depressed, because they are not appreciated, and then face the decision to move to another company, or risk the insecurity of striking out on their own (Levinson, 1977). Such decisions depend on basic characteristics that relate to childhood experiences as well as the individual's situation. Old sibling rivalries may have fostered a competitive attitude; a mother's expectations for achievement lead to a drive toward accomplishment; oral fixations lead to a need for security that interferes with impulsions to risk independence, etc.

The start of middle age is usually placed around the age of 40. For many, it is ushered in by several difficult years that have been termed the mid-life crisis or mid-life transition. The crisis is not set off by any significant event but rather by the realization that more time stretches behind than stretches before one. The balance of life is upset by awareness of the limits of life's span, and there is apt to be a recrudescence of existential anxiety concerning the insignificance of the individual life in an infinity of time and space. Two of the world's literary masterpieces start on this note. *The Divine Comedy* opens with the lines, "Midway in the journey through life, I found myself lost in a dark wood having strayed from the true path." Goethe's Faust finds that although he has studied philosophy, medicine, and law thoroughly, he is fundamentally no wiser than the poorest fool, and he makes a pact with Mephistopheles in an attempt to salvage something in life. At the start of middle age, there is still time to revise, time to start afresh, or at least to salvage the years that are left, but there can be no further delay.

The onset of middle age is commonly a time of stocktaking set off by the recognition that one's life is reaching its climax and may even have started on its way to its inevitable conclusion. Persons try to assess how their lives are going to turn out. Will dreams be fulfilled? Will life with one's spouse bring happiness and fulfillment? Must one come to terms with getting by? Or must one accept disillusionment and failure? However, the stocktaking concerns more than external success. It has to do with inner satisfaction and the hope of achieving a sense of completion and fulfillment. Are achievements compatible with one's ego ideal derived from early expectations? How great are the disparities between one's way of life and what provides a sense of self-esteem? For some, middle age brings angry bewilderment because neglect of meaningful relationships in the striving for success makes life seem empty. When, as sometimes happens, all goes relatively well in work and family life, middle age is a time of fruition, when the strivings and efforts of earlier years are producing tangible rewards. Most persons are now at the height of their potential, and even though they may have passed their physical prime, they can use their heads effectively and have learned to conserve their energies. They know their areas of competence and feel in control of them. They have moved to center stage, and assume responsibility. Some enjoy the prestige and power and they are impelled to seek after more power over others, but the sense of mastery in itself provides pleasure to less driven individuals. Truly successful persons have not simply acquired power, knowledge, and skills, but also wisdom in making decisions, approaching tasks, and in working with others.

For some, the years between 40 and 55 involve intense striving to catch the golden ring on the merry-go-round—to capture top positions or to climax a career by gaining the prestige or wealth that seems within one's grasp. However, many with their parental functions virtually completed are now likely to find gratification in a different type of generativity. They can now become mentors seeking to develop heirs in their fields of endeavor who will carry on their teachings and interests. They become involved in the future of the firms, universities, towns—the institutions in which they have invested their interests and energies. They sponsor persons who have the abilities to become their successors, or who will carry on their orientations. Erikson (1950) has considered generativity the crucial aspect of middle age, with stagnation the negative outcome. Stagnation comes with falling into a rut or routine, no longer seeking to learn and grow, or from disillusionment at not being appreciated, or perhaps, through lack of interest in anyone or anything beyond the self.

Although life for most will continue along the well-established path with satisfactions found along the way, disappointments absorbed, ambitions tempered by experience, concerns countered by religion or philosophy, various problems are likely to arise as persons cross the crest of life. The need for narcissistic reassurance concerning potency, attractiveness, or a longing for affection leads to a final fling before the closing of the gates. It may be a fling that can disrupt a reasonably satisfactory marriage, or sabotage a career. A marital relationship that had been maintained "for the sake of the children" is often terminated now that the children are adolescents or young adults, leaving one partner very much alone. Remarriage in middle age can work out well for those who have matured and can use better judgment than they did as inexperienced and impetuous youths; but a large number end up with a second spouse with basic characteristics very much like the first. The late 40s or 50s has often been a difficult time for women because of the menopause with the accompanying vasomotor instability and because of fears of an accompanying depression or the belief that it marks the end of active sexuality. Endocrine therapy can alleviate or eliminate the discomforts and the fears of emotional instability are unwarranted. However, the menopause often brings a transitory letdown as the woman loses her "badge of femininity." There may be an upsurge of sexual interest and enjoyment when pregnancy is no longer a concern, and women usually maintain more of their sexual capacities than men.

The "empty nest syndrome" may trouble women, particularly those whose lives have centered on their children, as they no longer feel needed and miss having children dependent upon them; but many mothers welcome the greater freedom and move into new vocations or avocations. The end of active parenthood can bring notable changes in the lives of both spouses as their freedom increases, but it can unmask difficulties between a couple now that their lives center on one another to a greater degree.

Health problems may interfere with the lives of the middle-aged. The body no longer responds without creaking or aching. Men are aware that heart attacks between the ages of 40 and 50 are particularly dangerous and can bring sudden death or incapacitation. Women check their breasts regularly for masses and have semiannual gynecological tests to detect the most common malignancies early. Obituary columns are scanned for the names of friends and acquaintances. Potential ill health and death consciously or unconsciously begin to influence their lives.

One of the critical aspects of middle age concerns coming to terms with one's accomplishments and future potential—not only to accept the limits of achievement and not become embittered and depressed over inadequate recognition, but also to be able to enjoy the prestige attained and to accept the responsibilities that accompany it. Not all can gain satisfaction from accomplishments if they are not rewarded or find pleasure in what they have made of themselves unless others appreciate what they have become. Even a promotion can bring trouble in the form of a "promotion depression." A man feels guilty because he has surpassed his father or father surrogate, reawakening old oedipal fears of paternal vengeance, and the man punishes himself for his hubris. Others, after gaining the desired promotion, resent the burdens of new responsibilities at a time when they no longer feel up to the new expectations and pressures.

As noted, the course of women's lives may differ markedly from those of men, particularly when they have gained renewal in middle age by starting on new careers. They may feel that they have already been fulfilled in life by having raised children successfully and although they pursue a new career with interest and devotion, their sense of worth does not rest so fully upon it as it does for the man.

OLD AGE

Just when old age starts has always been a rather arbitrary matter. It varies from person to person, but currently in the United States a rite of passage clearly marks the moment. Shortly before the sixty-fifth birthday, the individual makes a visit to the Social Security office and presents a few documents to establish qualifications for future social security benefits. Although the visit is brief, polite, and painless, those who make it are likely to experience a slight inner chill for they have now become senior citizens. Persons now begin to measure time in terms of years left rather than in terms of years lived. Aware of their decreasing earning capacities or depending on retirement pay, and cognizant of the precariousness of their health, income and health care become major concerns. Almost 40 percent of women entering old age have already had to make major readjustments when their husbands died. As only 10 percent of men are widowers, the disproportion between women and men becomes a notable factor in the social lives of the aged. Those who enter old age, however, are a somewhat select group. Life expectancy for men is still 13 years and for women 16 years, but they know that they will be fortunate if the remaining years are relatively healthy and untroubled and they can escape becoming unduly dependent before they die. For many persons, little has changed significantly and the crucial transition will come at the time of retirement, or for the housewife at the time of her husband's retirement.

Erikson (1959) has designated the achievement of integrity as the critical task of old age: the acceptance of one's one and only life cycle and of the people who have become significant to it as something that had to be and that, by necessity, permitted no substitutions. Integrity requires the wisdom to realize that there are no "ifs" in life; one was born with certain capacities, a set of parents, into specific life circumstances, in a particular time in history, encountered various conditions, and made numerous decisions, and so forth. Whether any of these circumstances could have been changed is questionable but the past cannot be altered though one's attitudes toward the past can be. The negative outcome of this stage of life is despair—despair that the one and only lifetime has been wasted leading to bitterness toward others or self-hatred that precludes the constructive uses of the experiences of a lifetime. Now persons are moving toward completion of the life cycle. Some feel that they are left standing at the end of the line with only a void before them, but others seek to bring a sense of closure to their lives and make efforts to round out what they have accomplished. In so doing, many elderly persons review where they have been, a process that may keep some persons rather fully occupied, but others are still achieving or helping others on their way. There is usually time for leisure and many will enjoy the leisure as an acceptable reward for their many years of work and striving.

In a sense, the aged person goes through a reversal of some critical aspects of adolescence (Lidz, 1976). The force of the sexual drive diminishes and much of the elderly person's sexual strivings come from desires for affectionate and sensuous sharing, much as in childhood. Then, as women lose the subcutaneous padding that rounded their contours and their secondary sexual characteristics, and men's musculature lessens, physical differences between the sexes diminish. Instead of being future-oriented, the aging increasingly turn to the past and what they have accomplished and experienced rather than to what is still to come. They will again become increasingly dependent, but now upon their children or others of the succeeding generation, which sometimes means that they must again become virtually obedient to caretaking persons lest they be rejected, as in childhood. Then, too, whereas adolescents move toward sharing their lives intimately with another, the aged must sooner or later absorb the loss of the person with whom they shared their lives. Nevertheless, early old age is autumn, not winter, and properly a time of contentment and a gathering of harvest.

The lot of the aged has, of course, been greatly improved over the past half-century by advances in medicine and various inventions. The electronic hearing aid has greatly diminished the proportion of elderly whose social lives had been blighted by deafness; cataract removal restores vision for many; dentures not only permit the enjoyment of food but reduce the incidence of nutritional defects. The automobile, radio, and television enable those whose physical abilities are limited to remain in touch with the world and enjoy entertainment. Nevertheless, the aged have less place in society than in former times as knowledge of the uses of the past is valued less in a rapidly changing technical society, and the young surfeited by television, cinema, and watching sports have little time to listen to the tales of the elderly and to learn to value what they have learned in a long lifetime. The isolated nuclear family often has little space or place for the elderly, though, as always, close bonds are apt to form between children and grandparents.

The elderly remain essentially unchanged from those in the middle years except for the difference in the way of life that may be created by retirement. "Being retired" may be resented, whereas retiring may be welcomed. However, much of the resentment and distress of retirement has come from the accompanying relative or real poverty. Those segments of the population with good financial provisions for retirement are likely to welcome it, happy to be free of the cares and monotony of work, and to have time to enjoy the many things they have put off and would still like to experience. Still, for many persons, old age goes best if there is still not enough time to do all the things one would like, if one is still caught up in a profession or the pursuit of an avocation. It is useful to remember that a number of gifted persons have reached the heights of accomplishment long after they entered old age: Titian, Matisse, Renoir, and Picasso produced some of their greatest works in advanced old age; Golda Meir and Winston Churchill were bulwarks of their countries long after most people retire.

When persons are fortunate and both members of the marital couple are still alive, their relationship tends to become increasingly important. Spouses not only care for one another but take care of one another, and hope that they will never need the help of any other. An upsurge of deeply felt and rather romantic love may occur. Contrary to the beliefs of the young, the elderly can, and often do, remain sexually active into advanced old age though the comfort of sensual closeness may become more important than orgasmic pleasure. However, sooner or later the invalidism of one partner brings the need for a major readjustment in the other. Life as a single person can be particularly lonesome for the elderly because of their limitations and loss of friends. Remarriage, or simply sharing life with a member of the opposite sex, has become increasingly common and acceptable and may bring real happiness to the aging person.

Advanced old age may be said to start at about the age of 75. Hopes for the years ahead usually have become modest as persons hope to find ways in which they still can be useful if not essential, but they are most concerned that they will not become a burden to anyone. Completing life in an old age home or nursing home, separated from family and friends, is a dreaded possibility. Those who enter advanced old age are a rather select group, for those who survive to 80 still have an expectation of living another 10 years and must plan accordingly. However, the majority become so limited by infirmities that they become dependent on the help and care of others.

Social relationships may become increasingly difficult to maintain as friends and relatives move away or die and infirmities restrict mobility. Retirement villages, sunbelt resorts and golden age clubs can help the aged find new acquaintances and keep active. Relatives, even those rarely seen since childhood, often become important as the ties of relationship permit visiting and common memories form bonds.

Some persons of very advanced age remain very vital despite some infirmities and manage rather full lives, utilizing their inner resources and making the most of what life offers to the end. Most persons who reach advanced old age, however, are, or will soon become, dependent on others. Dependency may be difficult to accept. Self-esteem based on self-sufficiency is undermined. Even when children are attentive, dependency can provoke frictions. Some old people react to needing help by becoming irritable or unduly assertive, whereas others can become a burden by pushing away proffered help.

Not all children are devoted to parents and some even gain satisfaction from dominating a parent who had once been dominating. Old people are rightly concerned about losing their autonomy, for when independence goes, individuality often follows.

All aged persons suffer a decrement in cognitive capacities. The fall is slight until the late 60s or early 70s, but even then, the loss is offset by the knowledge and skills acquired throughout life. Finding proper names becomes a common problem. A small proportion become senile and can no longer care for themselves. The most notable decrement is the loss of memory for recent events. It is as if a shade rolls down over the recent events until only memories of childhood remain. Individuals cannot guide themselves into the future, and eventually even routines become disrupted by faulty placement of the present into the remote past, and then a person requires supervisory care.

DEATH

Death brings the end of the life cycle, the inevitable outcome of the life story. Because humans from early childhood are aware of their ultimate fate, death influences their development and their way of life profoundly. Religions provide ways of denying that death is the final outcome, and utilize beliefs of what transpires after death as a means of controlling behavior. A large majority of persons in the United States believe in life after death, and some, in old age, attain a clear idea of what things will be like in a hereafter. Some old persons will cling tenaciously to life, but many have reached a stage where, deprived of those they love and limited in action if not living in pain, they are ready to welcome the Reaper who no longer seems so grim. Paradoxically, it is those who have never been able to really live because of their own neurotic limitations or because others have restricted them who fear death most. Yet, persons are almost always able to accept the inevitable. Those who do not wish to know that they will soon die usually have strong defenses against perceiving the obvious.

The efforts which are so commonly made to protect persons from knowing that they are dying often have unfortunate consequences. The dying often wish to discuss various matters that will concern those they are leaving, but a wall of deception separates the dying from family and friends just when they wish to be particularly close. Some do not wish to be deprived of experiencing that last experience they have often wondered about. Those who have gained wisdom in old age have usually ceased fearing death and may welcome it as a relief from the tribulations of life, particularly when those who have made life meaningful for them have already died. They are consciously or unconsciously aware that life is nature's greatest invention and death her means of making much life possible. How persons die and how others treat them in dying will affect those who follow as the experiences of one generation are handed on to the next.

REFERENCES

BENEDEK, T.: Parenthood as a developmental phase: A contribution to the libido theory. *Journal of the American Psychoanalytic Association*, 1959, 7:389-417.

BOTT, E.: Urban families: Conjugal roles and social networks. *Human Relations*, 1955, 8:345-384.

ERIKSON, E. H.: *Childhood and Society*. New York: W. W. Norton, 1950.

ERIKSON, E. H.: The problem of ego identity. *Journal of the American Psychoanalytic Association*, 1956, 4:56-121.

ERIKSON, E. H.: Growth and crises of the "healthy" personality. *Psychological Issues*, 1959, 1 (1), (Monograph 1).

JUNG, C.: *Psychological Types: The Psychology of Individuation.* (H. G. Baynes, trans.). New York: Harcourt, Brace & World, 1965.

KENISTON, K.: Youth and its ideology. In S. Arieti (Ed.), *American Handbook of Psychiatry*, Vol. 1. New York: Basic Books, 1974.

LEVINSON, D.: The mid-life transition: A period in adult psycho-social development. *Psychiatry*, 1977, 40:99-112.

LEVINSON, D. J., with DARROW, C. N., KLEIN, E. B., LEVINSON, M. H., & McKEE, B.: *The Seasons of a Man's Life*. New York: A. A. KNOPF, 1978.

LIDZ, T.: *The Person*. (Rev. ed.). New York: Basic Books, 1976.

Chapter 3

The Post-Parental Years:
Clinical Problems and
Developmental Possibilities

David L. Gutmann

While recent theoretical expressions in gerontology have paid lip service to the idea of a developmental psychology of aging, and entertained the possibility that personal growth can go on in the middle and later years, the conventional wisdom concerning the psychology of the second half of life is dominated by conceptions of loss and deprivation. Development implies a predictable addition, the emergence, in proper season, of hitherto unavailable potentials for new executive capacities. But our psychology, save for a recent statement by Riegel (1977), sees aging, starting in mid-life, as a period of continuous and irreversible losses. Thus, almost every recent text on the life cycle has a last chapter titled "Aging and Death."

In effect, the person transiting mid-life, or moving into old age, is almost invariably seen as a victim, defined and understood in terms of irretrievable deprivations. These presumably occur in all major spheres of existence: They are somatic, involving losses of health, virility, and fertility; they are social, involving losses of friends, older kinsmen, and children—the "empty nest"; and they are existential, involving the introduction to mortality, the "loss of future," and the loss of what Levinson and his colleagues (1978) call "the dream."

True, social scientists may differ as to the major source and nature of these losses. Thus, psychoanalytic theorists see the losses of later life as being traumatic not in themselves but because they resonate with and revive the traumatic losses of early life, while more traditional gerontologists refer to sheer quantity: Losses, they say, would be troubling in any season, and they are *concentrated* in later life. But whether they respond to the quantity of losses or their quality, psychoanalysts and gerontologists would see loss and deprivation as the central themes of aging.

Granted, losses *do* pile up in later life, but, by the same token, the likelihood of certain grievous losses recedes: Young men are much more apt to die in battle than old men—or of a broken heart. Some diseases, such as leukemia, carry off the young much more quickly than they do the old. Furthermore, while the aged are indeed more prone to particular losses, there is growing evidence that they do not feel them as keenly as younger people: Thus, the young are apt to treat death as a personal insult, while older individuals—for whom death has been normalized by the death of parents, kin, and friends—accept it with a certain equanimity, and sometimes even with relief.

In addition to being buffered against losses that are more devastating to the young, the aged also have available to them pleasures and powers that the young cannot appreciate and enjoy. Thus, a cross-cultural review of the status and satisfaction of the aging makes it very clear that our deprivational bias is indeed parochial, and limited to so-called advanced and secular societies. Simmons (1945) has shown—and my own field observations bear him out—that the small, face-to-face, traditionalist folk society is also a participatory gerontocracy, where older individuals acquire special powers and privileges not because of prior accomplishments, but merely by virtue of getting old. In such societies, one does not find the disengagement from social behavior or social norms that, according to Cumming and Henry (1961), characterizes the aging individuals of our society. Quite the contrary: In the small, traditional groups, the older individual is the very embodiment and enforcer of the moral norms of the society, and an old man can bless or curse with a force and an effect that is completely unavailable to younger men of the same culture. In such societies, where older individuals switch their investment from production to ritual, disengagement is only a temporary way station, and not the final destination. It is a prelude to new beginnings, rather than the beginning of the end.

Disengagement, then, represents an abortion of the natural sequence of divestment and reinvestment; it is the rule in secular societies which do not provide the ritual track for later life reengagement, but it is not a universal template for development in later life. It should be noted, however, that exceptions to the above rule do exist. For instance, the secular society does maintain traditional enclaves in certain professional subcultures, such as teaching, medicine, and the law. In these sectors, the aged practitioner retains much of the mythic force to bless and to curse that he is granted in the folk society. Indeed, it is a remarkable but generally unremarked aspect of the Watergate drama that Richard Nixon was in large part brought down by the dedicated efforts of old lawyers and legislators, most of them in their 70s and even 80s. True, young muckraking journalists attacked Nixon first, but they were as much interested in building their own reputations as they were in defending the Constitution. By contrast, the old lawyers no longer had a career to build; and they even put themselves at risk by attacking a politically powerful and vindictive president. While young men could certainly blacken the President's reputation, it was only the old war horses who had the conviction, the freedom and, therefore, the power, to bring him down.

By the same token, the power of Joseph McCarthy was broken by Joseph Welch, an aging lawyer, in the course of the Army-McCarthy hearings. Welch anathemized McCarthy before the nation, and his curse was potent enough to bring about the demogogue's decline and fall.

In effect, then, the picture of the older person as someone composed of losses and disengagements is a cultural phenotype, rather than a universal genotype.

Observations such as these, tending toward the conclusion that new growth potentials can continue to emerge across the life span, have inspired my own research into the comparative psychology of middle and later life. While it is clear that new executive capacities can mature under facilitating social conditions, the developmental potentials of middle and later life can only be accurately identified through such comparative, cross-cultural work. When we study age changes in a single society, we cannot disentangle nature from nurture, developmental imperatives from the social circumstances in which they are enacted. Observed in only one culture, developmental causes can be misread as the consequences of social guidelines and pressures. Developmental imperatives can only be highlighted when we look across a band of widely disparate societies, varying culture while holding age constant. The regularities in the ordering and sequencing of individual lives that we then observe, despite the widest possible variations in social circumstances, can then logically be linked to developmental influences, to nature rather than nurture.

Some intrinsic, nonsituational dimensions of middle and later life have been brought into focus by my own cross-cultural studies among various preliterate and agrarian groups: the traditional Navajo of Arizona, the Lowland and Highland Maya of Mexico, and the Druze of the Middle East. Through the medium of open-ended interviews and projective techniques, I have generated data among the younger (age 35 to 49) and older (age 50 and above) men of these groups, with the aim of establishing the outlines of a developmental psychology of the second half of life.

My findings on psychological change in middle and later life have been reported in detail elsewhere (Guttmann, 1964, 1969, 1975). Mid-life changes appear to be developmental in nature, can result in personal growth, and occur in predictable sequence across widely disparate cultures. We find that, by contrast to younger men, older men are more interested in giving and receiving love than in conquering or acquiring power. They are more interested in community than in agency. The younger men see energy as a feature of the self, as a potential threat that has to be contained and deployed to productive service. But the older men see energy as outside of themselves, lodged in capricious secular or supernatural authority. For older men, then, power must be manipulated and controlled for productive ends in its external form, through prayer and other forms of supplication and accommodation.

In sum, younger men tend to be businesslike; they do not go out of their way to seek pleasure, nor do they avoid any necessary work-related discomfort. Even their pleasures are mainly bound up with their work: They feel pleasure when they acquire control and mastery over the resources on which their security, and the security of their dependents, is based. Older men, by contrast, are more diffusely sensual, more sensitive to the incidental pleasures and pain of existence. Unlike the "phallic" young men, the older men seek pleasure in the pregenital direction: They become particularly interested not in what they can produce, but in that which is produced for them: food, pleasant sights and sounds, and uncomplicated, supportive human association. Where younger men look at the world instrumentally, and as an arena for competition and action, older men take some incidental bonus and aesthetic pleasure from their daily routine.

We also find, across a wide range of cultures, that women age psychologically in the reverse direction. Even in normally patriarchal societies, women become more aggressive in later life, less affiliative, and more managerial or political. Unlike the easygoing older men, they become less interested in communion, and more turned toward agency. Thus, over time and across sex lines, a massive trans-cultural shift seems to take place: During the post-parental years, the husband who used to support the wife both physically and emotionally now becomes more dependent on her; he tends to defer to her wishes and her requirements, acting toward her as he does toward other sources of security and authority in his life. In short, each sex becomes something of what the other used to be, and through these various gender changes, the normal androgyny of later life is ushered in.

In sum, it appears that both sexes reveal, in later life, the potentials that were blunted in the service of production, procreation, and parenthood. Thus, in their earlier years as young husbands and parents, men suppress those potentials within themselves—toward sentiment, dependency, sensuality, aestheticism, and even toward intimacy—that could interfere with their role as the productive parent, the provider of physical security. These dangerous, seductive promptings, that could prove lethal to their children, are sponsored in and lived out through the objects of their care, the wife and children who receive their nurturance. By the same token, the wife de-emphasizes her potential for aggression as it could interfere with her parental task—the provision of emotional security. As a colleague in child psychiatry put it, "If mothers did not suppress their anger, they would kill their children," and so young mothers learn to live out vicariously, through identification with the husband's exploits, the assaultive potential that could—if fully expressed—bring about the emotional crippling of vulnerable children, as well as the estrangement of the husband who provides for their physical security. Thus, during the active and critical period of young parenthood, each sex concedes to the other that aspect of their sexual bimodality that could interfere with their special responsibility in parenting. The transfer of psychic materials by each sex across the marriage bond is the equivalent, on the psychological level, of the transfer of genetic material on the biological level: Both forms of transfer are required to create children, and to keep them alive.

The prolonged period of emergency that we call parenthood requires another great transformation on the part of both parents: The transformation of narcissism into idealization of the child. Prior to parenthood, there is a tendency for the young individual to assert his or her right to maintain and nourish all aspects of self—even those that are mutually exclusive. Following the onset of parenthood, both parents give up the claim to omnipotentiality, and concede it to the child. In effect, the child's sense of basic trust, vital to healthy psychological development, pivots on the fact that the parents have idealized the child, and that they are ready to surrender their personal claim to centrality, to omnipotentiality, and even to life, in the child's favor.

The three great transformations—of communalistic needs, of aggressive needs, and of narcissistic needs—on which successful parenthood is based, are to some degree undone as children grow up and demonstrate, via their physical maturation, and by becoming mates and workers in their own right, that they can provide their own physical and emotional security. As the chronic sense of parental emergency phases out, there is less rationale on the part of either parent for maintaining the massive and energy-consuming repressions that are required by parenthood. As a result, a universal "return of the repressed," takes place in both sexes in which the psychological structures established and maintained by men and women in response to the parental emergency are, in effect, dismantled. The general consequence of this period of mid-life, post-parental relaxation, is the notable reversal of sex roles that we have observed in our transcultural data. For both men and women, there is, in effect, a return to the condition of pre-parental sexual bimodality: Both sexes in effect insist on their title, temporarily given up during parenthood, to be both male and female—to be omnipotential.

This demand, to be all-including, is essentially narcissistic. In the post-parental years, the narcissism that was once directed outward toward the vulnerable child now returns to reinvest the self, and the demand to be all-including is restated. The post-parental period of life—though its age of onset varies by culture and by social class— marks the point at which the three great relational modes—communalistic in the case of men, aggressive in the case of women, and narcissistic in the case of both men and women—once suppressed in the service of production and parenthood become available again to the personality, to become the pivot of renewed growth or of psychopathology.

In men, the potentials that are released by the ending of parenthood can become part of a new and heightened appreciation of the aesthetic aspects of life: Older men can become more aware of the incidental beauty of things, they can become more appreciative of children and of people generally, and they can become more religious —they may turn the feminine aspect that was once lived out through their wife toward the love and service of the gods. By the same token, women can discover in themselves an executive and "political" capacity that had hitherto lain fallow, and unrecognized: Formally or informally, they can play a domineering role in the home or in larger spheres that had once been closed off to them. Alternatively, they can identify themselves with the career of an ambitious son, the outward homologue of their own nascent masculinity: Where they once identified passively with the husband's career, they now fight actively, the power behind the throne, to advance the career of some favored young man.

In the post-parental period, children may still be loved, but they are less likely to be idealized: They have demonstrated their limitations, and their differences from the parents. Having taken a distinctive form, they have also acquired boundaries; they are no longer metaphors of the formless future with its multiple possibilities. Accordingly, new "objects" are required to bring about the later life transformations of narcissism that are required if the older person is to avoid a potentially disabling degree of egocentricity. The required object is no longer concretely personal—e.g., it is no longer a child—but generalized and social; thus, in traditional societies the older person can idealize the ritual system, as well as the gods and icons that sanctify this system. The aged link themselves to the gods and to the sacred practices, and thereby acquire a new source of self-esteem—one that is no longer based on their own productivity or procreativity, but, rather, on the potency of the gods with whom they are now, through ritual, merged. Men move from their younger location on the physical perimeter of the community to occupy a new niche on the spiritual perimeter, where they become a bridge between the pragmatic, daily community and the gods. Because they can idealize, they are also idealized by their community; and the aged of traditional societies take on, as we have seen, an awesome presence in the eyes of younger individuals.

A culture that provides proper collective representations at the proper season is thereby providing the psychological objects that allow for healing transformations and self-transcendence in later life. The potentially debilitating narcissism of later life is thereby transformed into the idealizations that sustain self and society. Instead of idealizing his own history, the older traditionalist can idealize the mythic origins of the whole society; instead of idealizing his own fussy, compulsive rituals, he can idealize the collective rituals that bind him and his community to the gods; and instead of demanding omnipotentiality for himself, he can idealize the all-powerful, all-including gods. From this vantage point of self-transcendence, death loses it personal sting. What is important is not the persistence of the self, but the persistence of gods and the proper life-ways that reflect their mythic nature. The special serenity that we call the wisdom of the aged is a by-product, a fallout from such fortuitous age-graded transformations.

When transformations of narcissism fail, when the collective representations do not appear on schedule, then both sexes may suffer a mid-life crisis of egocentricity, such that emeritus parents may become, in effect, their own children. Men in later life may express their self-concern through the passive mode, demanding the right to be cared for, while women might express egocentricity through the active mode, insisting on the right to be in total charge of their domain. For both sexes, the heightened self-concern can take the form of pettiness, irritability, and hypochondria: The digestion, the bowel movements, the articulation of the limbs can all become sources of fascination to the older person, if not to his audience. Endless reminiscence is another possibility, as the older person, unable to dramatize his present depleted self, seeks self-confirmation in an idealized personal past. This perspective is often escalated into a world view: The present, that belongs to the young, is full of weakness and corruption, and only the past knew true virtue and heroism. Unfortunately, the self is reinvested precisely at the time when it is most prone to suffer losses in the cosmetic, cognitive, physical, sexual, existential, and social spheres, and these losses are experienced by the egocentric elder as personal defeats and insults, rather than as natural (if painful) decrements. Too often, the sense of insult is warded off through desperate means: The idealization of the omnipotential, illusioned self is maintained through hypomanic denial of the blemish, or through paranoid projection of the imperfection onto others. The alcoholism that proliferates in later life in many cases plays the same function, of buttressing denial, and of filling the drinker with a temporary, hectic sense of his own omnipotence. Profound depression results when these quasi-psychotic defenses fail.

Unfortunately, modern psychiatry focuses on the losses of the older person, which are irreversible. The emphasis is on coming to terms with or medicating the pain of irretrievable loss. Practitioners would do better to treat the heightened but potentially reversible narcissism that renders these losses so poignant, so insulting, and so destructive. The emphasis should not be on resignation and adjustment to object loss; rather, it should be on guiding the patient toward forming those new and narcissism-transforming objects, the collective representations, that are appropriate to the post-parental season of life.

What is true for narcissism is also true for the other great relationship capacities that are released by the phasing out of parenthood. Thus, while many men can accomplish the transition to a more bimodal phrasing of their sexuality, and find therein an expansion of self, other men—much like adolescents—are frightened by the emergence of a new side to their sexual nature. This is particularly true in a society which, like ours, puts particular value on an uncompromised *machismo*. Like any stranger, the strange component of self excites, as it emerges, an initial fear, and in our *macho* culture, a sense of shame. Accordingly, we would predict that mid-life psychopathology, particularly in those men who have become troubled for the first time in the middle years, would be formed around threats from the "feminine" side of self.

This tentative formulation is borne out by preliminary work. Thus, a review of the cases followed in the short-term psychotherapy project of the Tavistock Clinic (London) indicates a significant shift, occurring after age 40, in the nature of presenting complaints and diagnostic formulations. We find that the younger Tavistock patients are mainly troubled by "Oedipal" issues, having to do with the inhibition of "masculine" sexual and aggressive strivings. The typical formulation for men under 40 sees them as victims of an unresolved struggle with a domineering father. The crippling guilt and anxiety that are aroused by this struggle lead the younger man to inhibit the aggressive and sexual strivings that have compromised the relationship with the father. A fair number even become impotent or homosexual in order to deny their "manly" but guilt-provoking urges. However, beginning around age 35 (particularly for working class men), there is a decided shift in the types of presenting complaints and diagnostic formulations. Older men are less apt to complain of a castrating father than of a domineering and smothering mother. By the same token, the feared quality of aggression is no longer discovered in the self, but becomes a quality of the wife—thus, an external threat. At least half the older men complain about an overbearing wife.

The inner life problems of older patients are not focused around genital and aggressive needs, but around internal, "feminine" motives: Older men, much more than younger men, are troubled by their wish to depend on others, to get out of the rat race, or to cry. Clearly, where younger men are troubled by the pressure from "masculine" and phallic issues that demand to be lived out, older men coming for psychotherapy are troubled by unmet "feminine" and pre-genital demands.

These tentative results, based on a small sample, barely deserve the title of "findings," but they do conform to the diagnostic impressions we have formed of older patients (45 and older) without prior history of psychiatric hospitalization whom we have studied at the Institute of Psychiatry, Northwestern University Medical School. Typically, these male patients are from 45 to 60 years old and reasonably established in love and work. In the large majority of cases, the psychiatric crisis is precipitated by, or closely associated with, mid-life changes in the wife: She has become financially and/ or emotionally independent, she has become more assertive, and she has become less adoring. Close diagnostic interviewing reveals the extent of the threat, and some approaches for dealing with it. Typically, these are men with strong feminine identifications, usually formed around a strong mother, who was viewed as extremely competent (particularly when compared to the father, who was typically seen as absent, and/or ineffective).

These men have never truly separated from the mother, perhaps because they lacked a compensating sense of maleness and paternity. They have disguised their lack of autonomy through hard work, and through living out the maternal identification via a relatively compliant wife. However, normal mid-life developmental changes have brought the wife "out of the closet," and her newfound autonomy is experienced by the husband as a personal rebuff, a distressing separation from the "maternal" figure. In addition, because the newly assertive wife is less willing to live out the "womanly" aspect of the husband's psyche, he is confronted with his own sexual bimodality, and panic ensues, often taking the form of an agitated depression.

In these cases, the "losses" which trouble the husband—e.g., of his wife's submission and adoration—are founded in development rather than some primary deprivation: Our patients are responding, albeit disastrously, to a linked process of growth that includes themselves and their wives.

We know that the incidence of male alcoholism escalates in the middle years, and our clinical explorations with late onset drinkers again suggest the centrality of post-parental developments in this syndrome: Alcohol is very good at sponsoring defensive externalization of the sexual bimodality that is underlined, for men, by the psychic shift of later life. Thus, within the course of the same drinking bout, the alcoholic is both a god and a helpless infant. He may start the evening by claiming that he can "lick anybody in the house," but he ends it in a stupor, unable to walk, and submerged in his own mess. He has experienced omnipotence and impotence. Alcohol, under the excuse, "it's the liquor talking," has taken responsibility for both of these extreme and mutually exclusive modalities.

Following the post-parental shifts in the domestic balance of power, psychosomatic illness can also serve—though at a great price —to restore the marital status quo ante: Thus, for the husband, a damaged organ can take on the role of the weak, dependent "feminine" entity that was once played by the wife. The patient approaches the doctor saying, in effect, "My spirit is strong, but my heart, liver, or stomach is weak," and petitions help not for himself, but for the organ for which he bears no moral responsibility.

The developmental perspective on such patients indicates a useful therapeutic as well as diagnostic line. The task in such cases is not to focus on the external counterparts and metaphors of loss, but again, to focus on the internal losses of self-esteem that come about as men—following the wife's "masculinization"—are forced to acknowledge the hidden "woman" within themselves. The therapist's task in these cases is to help these patients come to terms with this newly discovered aspect of themselves, so that their own "maternalism" can become a resource rather than a threat, and so that they can build new executive capacities, and new routes to pleasure, out of these possibilities.

The Tavistock sample of older female patients is too small to permit reliable judgment as to age changes in the sources of feminine psychopathology. However, it does appear to be the case that younger women, under 35, come to treatment in the "masochistic" position, complaining that they have been abused by others (and that they have permitted this abuse), while older women are more apt to be in the "sadistic" position, in that they are fearful of what they might do to others.*

These tentative results are consistent with the "developmental" hypothesis, and with our own clinical experience with first-admission older women patients. Thus, we predictably find that the typical diagnostic label attached to women in their late 40s and 50s is "depression," and the symptoms associated with that category lead automatically to diagnostic assumptions based on the "loss perspective": The depressed patient is presumably suffering through the menopause and the loss of her procreative capacities, she is suffering from the "empty nest," and she is suffering the pain of widowhood. But intensive interviewing as well as analysis of projective test imagery yields another story: Just as in the case of men, the real losses are more apt to be internal than external, based more on losses of self-esteem, rather than on a loss of some external supports or beloved person. For example, consider the case of a woman, hospitalized for depression, who is diagnosed as suffering from a kind of preemptive mourning for a terminally ill husband. The patient has been going to school, and was soon to begin a post-graduate career. However, these plans were aborted by the patient's decision to stay home and nurse her dying husband. The couple had been close, and the diagnostic formulation presented the patient as suffering and depressed in anticipation of the husband's oncoming death. However, the projective test images were not centered on loss, but rather on fantasies of imprisonment, claustrophobia, and rage. In effect, the patient was enraged over her imprisonment in a nursing

---

* I am indebted for these keen observations to Dr. Margaret H. Huyck, of the Department of Psychology, Illinois Institute of Technology.

role, at a time when she was looking forward to a more expanded and self-expressive post-parental life. She was not suffering the pain of loss, but the pain of guilt and self-reproach: She could not forgive herself for desiring the quick death—the death that would free her to an expanded life—of a beloved husband.

Thus, while the threat may come in each case from a different quarter, men and women in mid-life are prone to a loss of self-esteem occasioned by the growth of internal potentials—achievement motives in the case of the cited patient—rather than the loss of external support. Clearly, in such cases, the therapist should not concentrate on the loss which is irreversible—and which is no news to the patient—but on the guilt which is both unconscious and reversible.*

There appears to be a "deep structure" in the human psyche, a universal which states that candidates for aggressive power must endure the assault of that power against themselves, before they can own it and deploy it outwardly. By the same token, women in many cases appear to be enduring their own anger, in the form of depression, before they can own it, enjoy it, and turn it to alloplastic uses. In many cases, the hospitalized mid-life woman can be seen as suffering a kind of token death in depression, as a prelude to her "rebirth" in a more active stance. The period of hospitalization can be seen as a kind of "lying-in," during which the patient, through much pain, gives birth to a new self.

At any rate, the more we consider these matters, the more it begins to appear that the psychology of the post-parental period of the life cycle is not accommodated by the loss and deprivation conceptions that dominate our field. A better model than "loss" would be that of uncertainty. "Uncertainty" is the umbrella term that we

---

* Besides illustrating the clinical usefulness of the developmental approach, our work with older female patients also gives us some concrete evidence that psychological development continues through the adult phases of the life cycle, and thus offers further support to the theoretical validity of our perspective. Specifically, we find that quite old women, hospitalized for the first time in their 60s and following a reasonably productive life, are almost invariably childless—and not always by choice. Their history indicates that full, mature separation from the mother had never taken place: Since they had not become mothers in their own right, they could not achieve some decisive detachment from maternal figures. Accordingly, they remain vulnerable—even in adulthood—to maternal deprivation, and their transient psychoses, occurring in later life, often follow the death of an aged mother or mother surrogate.

bring to adolescence, to the troubled teen-ager who faces an unclear future with a changing body and changing definitions of pleasure. These terms travel easily across the life cycle, from adolescence to the post-parental period. In both cases, uncertainty implies not disaster but crises: New developments, new emergences can lead to disaster or to growth, and the issue is still in doubt. It is the clinician's job to recognize the growth possibilities inherent in the older person's crisis, to clarify the irrational threats that these entail, and to thereby sponsor the possibility of good crisis resolutions.

REFERENCES

CUMMING, E. & HENRY, W. E.: *Growing Old: The Process of Disengagement*. New York: Basic Books, 1961.

GUTMANN, D.: An exploration of ego configurations in middle and later life. In B. Neugarten (Ed.), *Personality in Middle and Later Life*. New York: Atherton, 1964.

GUTMANN, D.: The country of old men: Cross-cultural studies in the psychology of later life. Occasional papers in gerontology, No. 5, Institute of Gerontology, University of Michigan—Wayne State University, April, 1969.

GUTMANN, D.: Parenthood: A key to the comparative psychology of the life cycle. In N. Datan and L. Ginsberg (Eds.), *Life Span Developmental Psychology: Normative Life Crises*. New York: Academic Press, 1975.

LEVINSON, D. J., with DARROW, C. N., KLEIN, E. B., LEVINSON, M. H., & McKEE, B.: *The Seasons of a Man's Life*. New York: Knopf, 1978.

RIEGEL, K.: History of psychological gerontology. In J. Birren and K. Schaie (Eds.), *Handbook of Aging Psychology*. New York: Van Nostrand and Reinhold, 1977.

SIMMONS, L.: *The Role of the Aged in Primitive Society*. New Haven: Yale University Press, 1945.

Chapter 4

Suicide in the Middle Years: Some Reflections on the Annihilation of Self

Stanley H. Cath

SUICIDES HAVE A SPECIAL LANGUAGE

One of the major challenges of the mid-life period lies in the realization of one's limitations and capacity to live, love, achieve, and create. Not surprisingly, a vast range of human responses, including suicide, is associated with these multiple realizations and multiple interpretations of these realities. Actual or imagined insults to intactness of body-self, or more insidious depletions of self, are often superimposed upon threats to intrapsychic stability. These experiences may converge on the individual who, with age, inevitably becomes more vulnerable to narcissistic injury. This chapter focuses on describing some of the aspects of ego or self vulnerability as they relate to the suicide-prone person during the mid-life period.

The act of suicide, defined as an act or incident of taking one's own life voluntarily or intentionally, especially by a person in the years of discretion and of sound mind (*Webster's New Collegiate Dictionary*, 1974, p. 1165), is often perceived with hostility, censure, and condemnation. Each person figuratively builds for himself, in relation to the cryptic topics of suicide and death, his/her own conceptual framework of beliefs, understandings and orientations (Shneidman, Farberow and Litman, 1970). It is generally assumed that lay people are terrified but fascinated by suicidal acts. But it is not uncommon for mental health professionals to develop a predominately negative countertransference or, if you will, an outright fear and hatred of suicidal patients. These reactions may, in part, reflect a simplified categorization of dividing suicides into two groups, rational and irrational, and thereby ignoring the complex multiple realities of suicidal patients. Careful examination will reveal that such a dichotomous view is not only inaccurate but potentially harmful to our therapeutic position vis-à-vis the patient. For instance, prior to her consciously determined and thoroughly successful suicide, Anne Sexton (1976) wrote a poem which provides an interesting illustration of the notion of multiple realities and rationalities. She wrote:

> *Since you ask, most days I cannot remember,*
> *I walk in my clothing unmarked by that voyage . . .*
> *then the almost unnameable lust returns.*
> *Even then I have nothing against life.*
> *I know well the grass blades you mention,*
> *the furniture you place out in the sun . . .*
> *Suicides have a special language*
> *like carpenters, they want to know which tools.*
> *They never ask,*
> *Why build?*

In this brief excerpt, it is apparent that we must take suicidal men and women at their word and attempt to understand their language. They speak from their own viewpoint, unmarked or unmoved by ordinary values. They may not be cognizant of time in our time frame, and they may possess an "unnameable lust" for death. Utilizing a value scale significantly different from the world in which most people live, by their personal definition, they may sincerely believe they are "building something." It is my contention that Sexton shares with almost all suicidal people who have gone before an unconscious belief that man is continuous or life is continuous with nonlife. Even if there is no nonlife, such acts, no matter how irrational, occur in response to a special language and need. We must examine how these feeling states are reached.

The research literature on suicide indicates that while women of all ages attempt suicide more often (the peak occurring in females after mid-life), the most thoroughly completed suicides occur in middle-aged, seemingly successful men (i.e., physicians, psychiatrists, college professors, business executives, etc.). As such, middle-aged men represent the most lethally determined in terms of successful annihilation of self. Within the context of the previous discussion on vulnerability, we are confronted with an interesting paradox: How and why is it in mid-life, when many dreams or expectations seem reached or reachable, that an already considerable ego strength fails to sustain the self? Why is it that the rational mature ego failed to deter self-destruction, especially if he or she had achieved so much? Not only does this paradox make suicide seem particularly wasteful of highly intelligent/talented people, but it is even more devastating than anticipated to those intimately involved. The survivors experience an earth-shattering blow to their sense of ongoingness, to their ideals, to their wish for things to remain unchanged and to their faith in self-object constancy. At some point in time they raise the question: How can those who claimed to have loved us, shared our reality, and faced the same unpredictable future abandon us to an even more uncertain unknown? What was so bad about our shared reality, about us, about them? What was so frightening? We didn't see it that way. Were we such a burden? Does the same self-destructive tendency exist in all of us? Why do some people do it? Why not others?

It is my contention that it is the *quality of internalized long-past object relationships rather than success or failure of the immediate self-object relationships which determines the mid-life suicide potential.* I do not intend to deny the importance of environmental pressures or the individual's capacity to tolerate real life when it is objectively unbearable, but to emphasize the triggering rather than the etiological role others play in precipitating suicidal behavior. Within this context, suicide reflects past intrapsychic deficits in the investment of the self in others and as a result there is a reproduction of that flaw in the ego-ecological system as a significant holding environment. It is acknowledged that some suicides can be considered to be the result of a particular tension point which although fleeting was obsessively lethal. Still, it is the purpose of this chapter to focus on those whose self-intended suicidal acts are so incurably lethal that nothing we do over a long period of time, including the best efforts of suicide prevention centers, hospitalization, appropriate medications, etc., can stem the tide. Just when we believe these patients are improving or possibly cured, a well-planned lethal event will jar us out of such illusions. Let us assume that in every doctor's practice, there exist a few highly prone suicidal patients. Some repeatedly threaten but have no plan and never attempt suicide, while others may have a very secretive but well-thought-out strategy for the killing of the self when and if something may be interpreted as intolerable to the idealized self-image. A dreaded illness, which actually threatens real ongoingness of self, or a minor psychic insult, which only destroys the sense of ongoing perfection, may be equally lethal.

TRAGIC VERSUS GUILTY MAN

Kohut (1971) conceptually differentiated tragic man and guilty man, with the latter being a person in conflict but with a cohesive self while the former is a person prone to narcissistic injury. Clinically, serious contemplators of suicide, in my experience, tend to be clustered in an excessively sensitive, particularly vulnerable cohort of people for whom real loss or fantasized injury to self-esteem threatens basic self-cohesiveness and continuity of the perfect self. It is because of the depth of such vulnerabilities that ordinary events or anticipated injuries to the self trigger suicidal acts in the vulnerable cohort of the tragic man.

If it is true that the middle years of life may represent a time in which disappointment in self and self-objects is extremely intense, then it is necessary indeed to come to terms with sensed limitations of self-aspirations, or "time left" to achieve one's goals. A clinician must evaluate each individual's unique coefficient of anxiety related to aims, ambitions, and actualized realizations. He must study ego strength as manifested by a tolerance for loss and characterological responses to depletion and depression. These are balanced by the healthy storehouse of narcissism as it relates to "coherency of self," in order to comprehend the concept of the vulnerable cohort of tragic men.

The reader is referred to the works of Kohut (1971), Kernberg (1967), Mahler (1963), Spitz (1945), Greenacre (1971) and others to appreciate how psychological survival in later years depends on the very early presence of a responsive, empathic surround which allows a cohesive nuclear self to be formed. Mature selfhood, associated with the potential for conflict (i.e., "guilty man") is achieved by a process of internalized experiences derived from the earliest images and core-affective states. These early experiences involve safe infantile mirroring and merging relationships that provide a real sense of early significance, omnipotence and even grandiosity, leading eventually to the gradual establishment of an early sense of self in reality with reasonable entitlement and the capacity to bear frustration and disappointment. To accept the budding grandiose exhibitionism of a child contributes to a core or storehouse of self-sustaining narcissistic energy which may be called upon in times of stress.*

Faith in idealized self-objects, based upon the past security of daily safe mergers with an omnipotent other, carries us when in conflict, whether elated or in despair. For many middle-aged persons, no matter what happens to them, there remains this sensed promise of ongoingness, a caring closeness, which even in crises gives a feeling of calmness. Thus, a bulwark of a solid/integrated self is available to call upon when there are difficult losses to endure. The integrity of this inner calming "system" may be challenged or reinforced by the relationships one has created or by the utilizable social networks in the surrounding matrix.** *Therefore, it is not usually a single*

---

* If a child's parent suicides before age seven, the likelihood of suicide doubles, so that a suicidalist may well have been the victim of a previous suicidalist's attempts, failures or successes in the act.

** There may even be a biological base to man's self-soothing system, suggested by the recent discovery of "endomorphins."

loss, a momentous event or set of circumstances which overwhelms an individual, but rather his nuclear preoedipal character which determines his tolerance and ability to cope with the vicissitudes of life.

Even if one tends "to turn aggression in," the more one has experienced a mature empathic parental-self in tune with one's changing needs, the more one can protect the self from destructive urges, if indeed they are triggered when frustration is experienced. One can refuel the self and self-esteem either from within or by requesting reasonable gratification from significant others. The more parents can glow in response to their child's behavior and achieve gratification through the child, the more the child—grown adult— can activate some worthwhile grandiosity for himself from within when limitations and frustrations occur. *I would maintain grandiosity must be allowed a certain leeway early-on as a prerequisite for adult survival.* Yet one must also be able to curb excessive reactions and limit over-stimulation, to provide a sufficiently calm ambiance in the face of catastrophe, illness or death. While we have not always known how to differentiate "normal" dreams, ambition, and a healthy storehouse of self-esteem from grandiosity and certain forms of pathological narcissism, we are beginning to learn. We know that there are some who fragment under the stress of unreachable ambitions and disappointed dreams but then use regressive patterns of coping. Diagnostically, they may be referred to as borderline, narcissistic character disorders or psychotic individuals.

Still there must be an even wider range of different qualitative and quantitative responses to various realities and existential dilemmas throughout various lifetimes, leading to more subtle self-destructive qualities. These may manifest themselves as extremes of hopelessness, emptiness and helplessness. Some people may believe, temporarily or over long periods of time, that their life is impossible and should be terminated. But, somehow they find strengths from their inner reservoir of healthy narcissism or from a psychosomatic retreat to transcend, overcome and reregulate self-esteem in order to survive. However, we have not answered the perplexing dilemma of when the temporary impoverishments or failures are unlikely to provide the necessary barriers against self-annihilation. Are there other characteristic residual faults or early failures in ego structure formation which distinguish "conflicted man" with reasonably intact structural components from "tragic man" with extreme vulnerability to suicide?

PRESTRUCTURAL DETERMINANTS

It seems likely that biological as well as natal and early postnatal determinants may play a role in an early predisposition towards self-destructive behavior. During the earliest months of life, Cain (1961) was able to differentiate a particular group of infants because of their tendency to turn aggression against themselves. Anna Freud corroborated this observation in her emphasis upon the general defense of "turning against the self" as a genuine instinctual process, one independent of the development of psychic structures. This characteristic of "turning against the self" is as old as the instincts themselves, or at least as old as the contest between instinctual impulses and their hindrances which are encountered on the way to gratification. To quote Anna Freud, "We should not be surprised to find these are among the very earliest defense mechanisms employed by the ego" (Freud, 1966, p. 46).

Cain observed self-attacking behavior as a clear response to pain evident in certain infants as early as six months of age. Such children manifest mild, vicious, explosive, torturing, specific, purposeful or aimless behavior against themselves. Self-attack was triggered by frustration, deprivation, loss of love, or the loss of the presence of love objects. Within the first year of life, jealousy aroused by decentering of mother's attention, or loss of a soothing comforter may bring about similar responses. At first, some children attempt to direct anger externally, but should this not be possible, they may initiate overt attacks directed against the self "even as the initiator." *Anna Freud had conceptualized this auto-aggression as prior to the development of distinct self,* and Cain's direct observations of children harming themselves confirmed the very early roots. Beres (1958) differentiated attacks upon the self, from attacks upon the body, from attacks upon the ego as initiator (attacks from a subdivision of psychic structure—the superego) and suggested the beginning of what we may now consider "intrapsychic war." These intrapsychic attacks, however, are not likely to occur until 18 months of age when the superego is generally considered to become a functioning entity. Animal behavior reinforces the theory that inwardly turned aggression appears earlier than is generally thought and may well be on some instinctual basis.

Spitz (1945) in his study of "hospitalism" observed weeping sadness, dejected expressions, loss of weight, and susceptibility to illness in children as young as ten months of age. Some reacted to separation by depriving themselves of their usual enjoyment of toys and food. He could not tell whether or not the infant experienced self-reproach. It seems that we can consider these early experiences and observations as potential precursors of suicidal tendencies, in that they may be involved in the initial building of, or failure to build, a storehouse of healthy narcissism and outwardly directed aggression. Still, children who turn aggression against the self bring on reactions from those who care for them which may reinforce their tendencies, not to mention feelings of inadequacy, hopelessness, strangeness, and unlikeability. Simultaneously, they effect a centering of attention upon their destructiveness, which becomes a central theme in their intrapsychic life and in their self-object relationships.

Thus, at the root of self-destruction may be very basic affective states linked to early core experiences of self-directed aggression which relate to a failure in formation of a self-confident, continuous cohesive self. Failures of empathy or in early bonding, suffered because of inadequate or unempathetic mothering, reinforce further failure in the capacity of self-calming and soothing which may be required in tense transition periods throughout life. These factors may be the ones which become the ultimate determinants of lethality in suicidal intents and acts. I would suggest that differentiation of intent from act is of limited value unless these earliest affect states are considered.

A NEW SYNTHESIS: THE WAR OF INTROJECTS

To illustrate the potential for deeper understanding leading to different therapeutic modalities, let us look at a parallel series of interpretations in which this conceptual framework is appended to that suggested by Shneidman (1976).

Let us begin by defining suicide as he does, as a self-intended and self-inflicted act with the purpose of cessation. It seems appropriate to ask, why has cessation become necessary? Cessation of what or rather of what part of the self? One may offer a different viewpoint: Namely, a suicidal tragic man has been in a relatively unchanging intrapsychic war involving past self-object introjects. The conflict is reinforced by a present or current appraisal of actualized "parts" of the self and in self-other relationships. Thus, "self-intended and self-inflicted" must be broken down into an active and passive part of the self. The passive parts have always needed to be changed but now deserve to be destroyed. *These parts or introjects are made up of a balance of multiple images, derived from past and present relationships, but which derive their major vitality from past affective qualities of earliest and more primitive loving and hating self-objects.* These hated or negative past introjects have been integrated into a somewhat imperfect, but still cohesive, whole, self-respecting, self-loving self. It is these hidden aspects of the alienated self which must be destroyed.

We might well ask if they could be tolerated before, at what point do they become intolerable? Several points are relevant here. It seems not enough early aggression was neutralized or transmitted (converted) into a storehouse of self-preservative forces. Rather, aggression was stored in moral strictures and intense, unforgiving, demanding perfection of self and others. When a developmental failure in transmuting internalization (the neutralizing and synthesizing of hating-loving self-objects into a single whole) is activated by a challenge to the illusion of omnipotent control over self or others, an enhanced split between good and evil is demanded. This enhanced splitting phenomenon cracks the ancient flaw. Such discarded, split-off, evil introjects then lead to the creation of a self-object world in which real objects (i.e. members of the family or therapists) become recipients of the split-off, despised aspects of the self. They are beyond reach—if one cannot control the external world, one cannot control the inner world. By projective identification, these negative images are intermittently attached to the selected person.* As a result, the family or therapist may become less real, less believed in terms of loving and caring, of providing a safe holding environment, and less capable of counteracting internalized negative images than might be expected. Thus, "loved ones" find it difficult to communicate with and convince a suicidal person of his worth, either to them or to himself, or of the true value of self-objects around him. This is partly because current objects have never gained ascendancy over past ones nor have they been adequately differentiated from the mental representations of hateful self-objects of the past. Survivors are left to puzzle why ordinary failures have triggered such rage and why the individual, himself, or his family as a representational part of himself, deserved the fate of ultimate and complete annihilation. No matter how rational such suicides may seem they are rarely rational to survivors. Indeed, some people who commit suicide carry others along with them in a mass destructive orgy which leaves little doubt about the mental representations and the projective identifications. *Cessation seems the only possible solution—cessation of the intrapsychic war between mental representations and projective identifications.*

While self-destructive states are usually linked to depression, I would point to the reconstruction of a *psychological triad, namely, depletion of loving energy, splitting of good and evil (fragmentation of self) and loss of cohesiveness.* This triad of tragic man lies far beyond the realm of depression (guilty man), and suggests that past failures in human empathy have resulted in extreme hopelessness. It is a failure of parental empathy which leads to the suicidal person's failure to empathize with his loving self and/or the surviving, "loving" self-objects. It is this triadic constellation which leads to ultimate lethality. We need, however, an enhanced awareness of how, why, where, and when a person enters such a state of altered consciousness in which timelessness, hopelessness and helplessness are so involved. Such differentiations are not to be found in either the usual textbooks or psychiatric classifications. It is this clinical issue which desperately needs to be addressed. States of in-

---

* One father suicided shortly after his teenage daughter "lived with" her boyfriend. He had consciously condoned this as "what everyone does these days"—but it represented an intolerable capitulation of a more serious nature on another level.

ternal, quiet, angry agony, or highly covert existential anxiety exist in far greater numbers and in much larger segments of our population than is generally assumed.

Shneidman's second obervation speaks to this quality of "inimical inimicability." From a psychoanalytic perspective, this may be considered a derivative of narcissistic rage from past narcissistic injuries, leading to splitting and depletion. We are dealing with a failure in the formation of sufficient ego structure to contain or neutralize the deepest infantile sense of "hurt"—leading to a desire for revenge.

His "perturbation," from this perspective, reflects a state of restless intolerance for the split-off affects of love and hate. This anxiety becomes apparent when the compensatory defenses which may have worked for a part of life are disrupted and basic personality flaws, hidden from view in the past, become manifest as "perturbation." Shneidman speaks of "constriction" or "single-mindedness." In my opinion, an actual psychophysiological shift in attention cathexis towards these past negative introjects leads to another level of consciousness. It is this constriction or shift in attention cathexis which distorts cognitive-perceptual processes. The distortion occurs as a result of the demands of the intrapsychic task of containing the extraordinary intensity of rage, the seemingly justifiable "self-hatred" as well as the urgent necessity of removing the offending parts of the offended self by annihilation. This becomes the tragedy of tragic man.

In short, Shneidman's concept of "cessation" represents the wish to annihilate hated parts of internalized self-objects with which one is too much identified. It is not a cessation of the total self, but only the split-off part of the hated self-object, which, in intrapsychic economy, must be put out of existence. We have still to encompass the complexity of suicidal man.

SUICIDAL NOTES AND SURVIVOR GUILT

Suicide notes, according to Shneidman, are often repetitive if not boring and banal. Certain themes echo and reecho over and over again. "It was the only path I could take. I have been so injured, I cannot stand the pain. In spite of everything, I want you to know I love you. Do not feel guilty, forgive me, I forgive you. Don't blame yourself, no one is to blame."

On a superficial level, it seems these notes have some merit in reference to why they were left, namely, to contact and comfort those about to be bereaved. Yet, they rarely do comfort and seem strangely reminiscent of a small child's response to anticipated criticism, or his attempts to undo guilt over contemplated aggression. They are in a way saying, " I am sorry, but I was too weak. Don't hate me too much—let me repair things a little!" We need to ask what is it that could not be tolerated and if it could not be tolerated, why is no one to blame? Did the individual recognize that he was dealing not only with an abnormal sensitivity in himself, but also with a reduced capacity to let others bind his wounds? How can he blind himself to survivors' guilt? He must know, inevitably survivors ask, "Who is to blame? What will I do with all my guilt?" Everyone involved, even friends, feels accountable. Let me suggest that the reason no one here and now is to blame, is because no one external to the self-object system has had that realistic or important a role. Another way of saying this may be an even greater blow to the self-esteem of survivors: Others had not been sufficiently cathected in reality, as to be able to play a significant life-saving part in neutralizing injuries based upon failures in past empathy. In brief, they could not lessen the severity of the long-established intrapsychic war, shore up the damaged self-esteem, diminish unconsciously stored-up resentment over past empathic failures, or stem the tide of revenge.

THE MID-LIFE TRANSITION

It is paradoxical that at the midpoint of life when one is confronted by a very personal meaning of aging through the aging and death of one's parents, one's own decline is counterpointed by the emergence, if not exploding into life, of sexuality and creativity in one's offspring. Most families experience these developments as a critical challenge of transition, albeit in slow motion. As a common heritage, the decades after age 35 contain at least three questions.

1. Why do I live, age, and relate in this way?
2. How much longer do I have to live at my best, or to correct my ways?
3. How will I age, with what human supports, and how will I die, . . . with integrity or despair?

Every reflective human being goes through a series of self-monitoring inventories and self-assessments (Cath, 1966), a life review, (Butler, 1963), a reassessment of goals (Gould, 1977). Ego ideals must change during these years as aims/ambitions of self and expectations of objects (and of mental representations of the transitional world) come into conflict with actualized reality. This balance is influenced by the interactional feedback sensed from others. An accumulating body of information, including disappointments in the self-object world, must be reconciled with grandiose expectations of what one feels should have been one's lot or what one still expects it to be. A related issue which persists during the mid-years is the tendency to rationalize that what one has chosen must have been correct and what one anticipated still must be valid and respected. Such narcissistic semi-delusions coexist side by side with the knowledge that choices and decisions were not always correct. Similarly, the demand for continuity of an unchanging self-object world contrasts with the awareness that certain significant relationships, such as marriage, may have changed dramatically over the years.

The task of comforting the self is enormous. The demand for perfection or the impossible, from self and self-objects, may persist in a last ditch stand, as if to scream out "my narcissism must be served." The paradox lies in how elements of grandiose expectation can continue to exist in the face of a world which one now knows to be imperfect and with full awareness that unless one distorts perceptions, the self-object world can only yield so much. The more one's character is permeated by certain narcissistic issues, of lifelessness, emptiness, craving for the relief of "centrality," the more difficult the shoals of the mid-years are to negotiate. There is a further complication based upon the need to reconcile oneself to a declining sexual image, determined often by a biological or organic "clock."

For some the realization of limited time left, shifting social mores, and limited energies available leads to a shift in values and goals. This may include either an intensification or an abandonment of career activities. The necessary confrontation with one's parents' aging and mortality may spur one's use of limited creativity or fertility. A "relicensure of self" (Gould, 1977), in regard to intimacy or deviancy permitted, may lead to a split in love objects (i.e., wife plus mistress) or a complete break of old partnerships and/or significant alterations in life-style. Such attempts to reinforce the "mid-aging-self" may include some reacceptance of previously rejected parts of the self (i.e., the dependent or nurturant sides), a move away from family toward a career (especially in women), or a reconsideration of previous choices to remain barren. But increasing appreciation of the inevitable depletion of self (i.e., the body and all basic anchorages) may lead to intermittent regressions with periods of confusion about object ties, ideals and goals. Intense wishes to separate one's self from one's past, to break from all bonds and restraints or to be reborn often suggest magical thinking. Thus, to preserve a sense of self-object constancy and ongoingness is a constant challenge in the mid-years for everyone.

MID-LIFE AND THE SUICIDALIST

Clinically, the mid-years are a time of intermittent loss, grieving, mourning, turning inward and efforts at restitution. The sequential disability and loss of parents, uncles, aunts, friends, or interrupted careers leave their mark on everyone. But to the narcissist and/or suicide-prone individual, the loss of an idealized useful or grandiose image of the self can be doubly accentuated via physical disability to the self or objects from whom one is not clearly differentiated (for example, a 50-year-old man became suicidal shortly after his daughter began living with her boyfriend, his son was picked up for shoplifting and his wife developed a degenerative nerve disease).

When restitutive efforts are not successful, psychosomatic way stations, fatigue and other regressive equivalents appear and become the concern of sensitive physicians or caretakers. In the face of physical handicaps or disease, the more mature will shift their value systems, so that physical intactness and strength will no longer possess such high priority. Rather, mature skills, judgment, and supportive understanding will replace the inevitable body failures or fill the personal voids we all endure, permitting an ongoing sense of purpose, control and lovingness. Still others act out their problems in more self-destructive ways. Some destroy what they have created (i.e., artwork, business adventures, etc.) or let themselves be exploited by quacks, or taken advantage of by grandiose manipulators. They seem to create misery by losing self-protective instincts. Through self-destructive judgments, they may commit occupational or financial suicide (i.e., embezzling funds as if in a panic to accumulate "reserves"). Others turn their back on those who might love and support them in the lean years ahead in a search for either an illusory ideal of youthful beauty or an elixir of youth. These attempts have a high social cost sometimes reverberating through generations, as they tend to destroy the faith in mature families, even if the individual does not totally destroy himself.

From one point of view, such defenses can be understood as adaptive protective maneuvers, but the total overall cost of self-destructive aspects of the mid-life crisis, individually and collectively, is enormous. By this time of life, every intimate loving relationship also contains its reservoir of hurt feelings and injured pride. By contrast, the more healthy middle-aged neurotic may try other defenses to repress anger and, in general, use "healthier" mechanisms than denial and splitting. The more disturbed attempt to cover their more serious "primary (earlier) defect" with polymorphous, perverse behavior, especially when confronted by a loss of the idealized, sexual, youthful self or physical intactness. Confusing the failing body self with total self may lead to wishes to give up the lease on life. Some, intolerant of imperfection and aging, prefer to die at their peak. From this disturbed perspective or in this language, the suicidal individual can see nothing worthwhile ahead.

So it would seem that in psychiatry and psychoanalysis, a historically justified focus on conflictual or "guilty" men has neglected the role of tragic men or narcissistically vulnerable men. Both family and therapist's countertransferences limit our ability to help such patients. Our responses to attempted self-destruction often reinforce the negative qualities of the self-image (i.e., this person is a coward, a moral degenerate, a deserter, etc.). Our understandable rage is reinforced by and mirrored in the patient, who often holds himself in equal contempt because of his fragile self-esteem and dependency upon others. This secret contempt is especially displaced onto wives who had been originally chosen to fulfill unconsciously sensed gaps in the husband's self, or to unrealistically cover over defects of his character.

In his paper on object choice, Freud (1948) suggested that people may choose someone as a nourishing protective object primarily to gratify infantile needs (i.e., the anaclitic form of object-relationship). Another form of object choice (mirroring) is someone designed to fulfill a missing part of the self (i.e., to mirror back a quality felt missing), for example, strength to cover a sense of inadequacy. In such cases, the relationships can be considered primarily "narcissistic," or self-completing. Such attempts to recapture idealized relationships or to replace missing parts of the self reflect an imperfect development of a cohesive self. Thus, the preservation of archaic self-object structures is characteristic of the suicidalist. In mid-life or later, when a spouse is lost, the self-object world of vulnerable people is experienced as shattered or fragmented. On occasion, such a loss precipitates direct or indirect suicidal behavior. Sometimes anaclitic relationships of the type described are threatened earlier when the person "chosen" matures into a person in his or her own right. This may be a result of therapy, or a series of serendipitous events beautifully illustrated in the Woody Allen movie, *Annie Hall*. The hero convincingly and sincerely urged his love object towards independence and growth. When she achieved a modicum of this independence, he could not tolerate the separate interests she developed, especially when she needed more than he could provide. Their relationship changed from an exclusive comforting one-to-one mode to the threatening inclusion of intruding others. Separation became inevitable as the unconscious symbiotic dyad could no longer be maintained. But some symbiotic relationships may be adequate to stock "the narcissistic cupboard" for a lifetime. In especially vulnerable people, the process of depletion characteristic of the 30s, 40s, and 50s begins to take a toll. There are many roads, then, over which suicidal persons and their families travel before they reach a final common path.

A TRAGIC MAN—FROM LITERATURE

The concepts discussed within the context of this paper are illustrated in a review by Shainess (1977) of John Cheever's novel, *The Swimmer*.

A middle-aged, wealthy, high society man decides on a seemingly amusing odyssey: to swim some eight miles through his neighbors' string of pools back to his home. While the story is initiated with the joie de vivre of a humorous lark, it soon develops into a tale of a "tragic man." His mid-life contained grandiose fantasies linked to an adolescent sense of immutable macho. The superficial veneer of success covers a vulnerable age-inappropriate, agonized but entitled self. The story suggests serious developmental failures which have led to both self-deception and poor adult relationships. But his reservoir of self-esteem does not seem overtly depleted and he does not commit suicide directly. Rather, he successively confronts and destroys many idealized representations of himself with which the story initially opens. It is left to the reader to decide whether or not he ends in total self-destruction.

Unable to readjust to middle age or appropriate ideals, "the swimmer" attempts to restore the adolescent dream of an exhilarating journey, of being loved by everyone and welcomed everywhere. He seemingly exhibits an eternally youthful, powerful, and sexual image. In the series of encounters in and around his neighbors' pools, we gradually become uncomfortably aware of the threatening qualities of his failure in transition into middle years. The story vividly portrays a loss of sensed continuity with a tenuous past, of connectedness with a fickle present and a terror of an unpredictable future.

First, he encounters a very young and beautiful girl in a bikini, a former babysitter of his children. After an initial impression of "love-making," the romance turns into a strained seduction and as her resistance is increased, to an overt attempt at rape followed by rejection. If we assume the author utilized the literary device

of inverting ages, this relationship reflects strong incestuous over-
tones. As a result, punishment would be expected and sure enough,
in their "sexual" struggle, the hero is injured. It is as if the scene
symbolically recreates the theme of oedipal transgression, which
leads to a tragic flaw. The swimmer must now proceed on his
odyssey with a twisted ankle as well as the narcissistic wound of
a deep sense of rejection. He limps onto the next pool, where an
older woman, after granting him another of his constantly requested drinks, reminds him of his nasty rejection of her after a
long past affair. Revengeful, she now orders him on his way. If too
much is assumed in thinking superficially of these encounters as
oedipal issues, the author suggests the even more childlike quality
by quoting: "He knew he had lost his golden playpen." At another
pool, the owner confronts him with another harsh reality—he is
accused of hypocrisy in his love for his children. Rather than being
proud of him as he always thought, his daughter is ashamed of
him. He limps on from pool to pool each time encountering a
confrontation more painful than the last.

Such confrontations in the mid-years lead to "inventories" which
call into account naive assumptions of the decades prior to the
mid-years, inventories which challenge our sense of continuity and
omnipotence repeatedly. Traditional success, the value of money, social position and prestige, the notion of growing upward and on-
ward are inevitably disrupted by recognition of common human
failures and vulnerabilities due to the passage of time. Cheever
makes many ominous references to time or confusion about time.
Metaphorically, the swimmer never knew what time it was nor
did he realize it was getting late or too late. When the stars of
winter came out (Andromeda, Cepheus and Cassiopeia) he began
to cry. Where were those of summer? In the mid-years, each in-
ventory reinforces the other in a form of convergence, contributing to a sense of limited time left. As in this "swimmer," wear and
tear, exhaustion, depletion and despair may seem concentrated in
body muscle. Symbolically this feeling of depletion may also represent an excessive mid-life preoccupation with physical capacity
needed to sate infantile demands for pleasure and for accomplishments. Such self-preoccupation ignores or suppresses the swim-

mer's lack of fidelity to ideals and to significant self-objects. As the story unfolds, his developmental arrest helps to explain why desperate loneliness, anxiety and isolation threaten to engulf both swimmer and reader. But still, he and we are buoyed up with hope.

The swimming path, the string of pools, was named the Lucinda River, after his wife. Even though he had repeatedly deserted her, it seemed to symbolize his residual hope that his marriage might still provide some form of safe continuity or a supporting stream of past, present and future. It was as if he was swimming back towards the headwater of that river. But in another regressive scene, he is forced to beg for a quarter and to enter a public pool. Like a child, his feet are dirty, and he is required to wash repeatedly before he can enter. Although exhausted, he can barely swim, he persists as if his continuing odyssey were of a life-or-death nature. Finally, after reaching home in a blinding rainstorm, he finds himself locked out, the windows broken and his home deserted. Empty, self- and objectless, with no one to love or to love him, he sinks in humiliating despair to the ground as if to die of exhaustion, depletion and exposure.

The Swimmer vividly portrays one kind of "tragic man," the one who "needs to swim in everyone's pool, to chase every woman, to drink of every neighbor's resources and to be a part of everyone else's life." But the analogy to suicide is more than suggested in the final scene when he sinks lifelessly to earth.

As psychoanalysts, we may talk about the narcissistic vulnerability of suicidal individuals and their fantasies about rebirth and restitution, of reunion or fusion with an idealized self-object, but still we may not communicate any more clearly than the poets. This presentation adds a somewhat technical attempt, another dimension, to what poet Anne Sexton and author John Cheever have done so eloquently. It contains the hope that better understanding may lead to better methods of intervention.

REFERENCES

BERES, D.: Vicissitudes of super-ego functions and super-ego precursors in childhood. *Psychoanalytic Study of the Child*, 1958, 13:342-351.
BUTLER, R. N.: The life review: An interpretation or reminiscence of the aged. *Psychiatry*, 1963, 26:65-76.

CAIN, A. C.: The presuperego turning inward of aggression. *Psychoanalytic Quarterly,* 1961, 30:171-208.

CATH, S. H.: Beyond depression—the depleted state. *Canadian Psychiatric Association Journal,* 1966, 11:329-339.

FREUD, A.: *The Ego and the Mechanism of Defense* (Rev. ed.). New York: International Universities Press, 1966.

FREUD, S.: Contributions to the psychology of love, a special type of object choice. *Collected Papers,* 4:192-202. London: Hogarth Press, 1948.

GOLDBERG, A. & KOHUT, H.: *The Psychology of the Self, a Casebook.* New York: International Universities Press, 1978.

GOULD, R. L.: Psychoanalytically based theory of adult development. Unpublished manuscript, 1977.

GREENACRE, P.: *Emotional Growth* (Vol. 1). New York: International Universities Press, 1971.

KERNBERG, O.: Borderline personality organization. *Journal of the Psychoanalytic Association,* 1967, 15:641-685.

KOHUT, H.: *The Analysis of the Self; a Systematic Approach to the Psychoanalytic Treatment of Narcissistic Personality Disorders.* New York: International Universities Press, 1971.

MAHLER, M.: Thoughts about development and individuation. *Psychoanalytic Study of the Child,* 1963, 18:316-324.

SHNEIDMAN, E. S.: An overview of suicide. *Psychiatric Annals,* 1976, 6:9-121.

SHNEIDMAN, E. S., FARBEROW, N. L., & LITMAN, R. E.: *The Psychology of Suicide.* New York: Science House, 1970.

SEXTON, A.: *45 Mercy Street.* L. G. Sexton and L. Conant, Jr. (Eds.). Boston: Houghton Mifflin, 1976.

SHAINESS, N.: The swimmer. *The Academy,* 1977, 21:13. Newsletter of the American Academy of Psychoanalysis.

SPITZ, R. E.: An inquiry into the genesis of psychiatric conditions in early childhood. *Psychoanalytic Study of the Child,* 1945, 1:53-64.

Webster's New Collegiate Dictionary. Springfield, Mass.: G. & C. Merriam Company, 1974.

Chapter 5

Psychotic Illness in Mid-Life

Malcolm B. Bowers, Jr., John Steidl, Deborah Rabinovitch, Jean Brenner, and J. Craig Nelson

This chapter will focus on the nature of psychosis occurring in mid-life, and for the purposes of this discussion we have defined mid-life as beginning at age 30. We have previously presented a model of psychotic illness which is derived from an analysis of clinical experience (Bowers, 1974). In accounts from psychotic patients, it seemed that we were able to identify different qualitative processes of form, content, and timing. The form of psychotic experience is the novel cognitive pattern that emerges as the syndrome develops. It includes the pace and pattern of ideational processes, the widening of consciousness in the emergence of unconscious thoughts, the broadening of categories of relevance, and the urgency for making sense of the experience. The content of psychotic experience, by contrast, is largely determined by individual experience. The specific subject matter or referents of the increased ideational process, the particular ideas that surge into consciousness, and the specific personal meaning that evolves are included in this category. The timing of the psychotic episode refers to the life stage and particular stressful circumstances surrounding the onset period.

From a consideration of the qualitative ingredients in psychosis, we attempted to identify the psychological processes or components which underlie these qualities. The first component we described is the so-called state component, that is, the psychotic state itself. This component refers to the various altered states of mental functioning and their objective and subjective phenomenology which are seen in the various psychotic illnesses during symptomatic periods. It is roughly equivalent to classical secondary symptoms in psychosis and to Axis I in DSM III. This component usually reflects the classical diagnostic terminology, e.g., schizophrenia, schizoaffective illness, manic-depressive illness, delusional depression, etc. The second component, a trait component, refers to those premorbid aspects of personality usually seen to one degree or another in individuals who develop psychotic illnesses. The clinical referents here are asocial behavior, tenuous social relationships and heterosexual bonds, and low energy or competence. The third component, which we will emphasize in this chapter, refers to factors related to onset of the psychosis and has two parts. The first part is the generic developmental phase the patient has reached. The second consists of the specific life stresses or challenges which are associated with the onset of illness. Dynamically, stresses associated with particular developmental stages are hypothesized to act upon premorbid traits and unknown biological vulnerabilities to produce a psychotic state. We have previously described a paradigm whereby each of these components of psychotic illness can be taken into account in a comprehensive treatment (Bowers, 1977).

We want to emphasize that we are not convinced that the stress component is the primary etiologic factor in these illnesses. Therefore, our ability to learn about normative mid-life in the study of these syndromes may be limited. Nevertheless, in the treatment of such individuals, one is usually left to work with these stresses and developmental issues in long-term therapy. Further, our own experiences suggest that the developmental issues which are associated with the onset of psychosis in mid-life are precisely those which we identify in normative development.

The study of these later-onset psychoses may have particular clinical relevance, for they do not include, for the most part, those schizophrenic illnesses classified as process or poor prognosis forms. Since the pioneering work of Leslie Phillips (1953), clinicians have known that the level of maturity prior to the onset of psychosis plays a major role in prognosis. Many patients who become psychotic in mid-life have achieved some degree of adult maturity and have some accomplishments in the development of intimate adult relationships. These individuals often seem to be workable in therapy and to be able to achieve even further growth.

As an approach to the study of these patients we have begun a retrospective investigation of 45 patients (8 male, 37 female) between the ages of 30 and 59 (mean 41.7) hospitalized for psychosis. Patients were selected for study if they had not been hospitalized before or if there had been clear periods of good functioning between hospitalizations. A majority of patients (67 percent) were married. Only 16 percent had never married. With regard to prior hospitalizations, 33 percent had none, 22 percent one, 20 percent two, 20 percent three, and 5 percent four or more. They had completed an average of 12.9 years of school. Two-thirds of the patients were living with their spouse. All patients were diagnosed according to Research Diagnostic Criteria (Spitzer, Endicott, and Robins, 1977). Using these criteria, the following numbers were obtained: schizophrenia, 5; schizoaffective illness, 2; mania, 10; delusional depression, 12; and other functional psychosis (usually a paranoid illness without Schneiderian first rank symptoms), 16.

Two approaches were used to understand the timing of psychosis in these patients. As noted, timing was felt to be determined by developmental phase and specific life stresses, and was analyzed by assessing the life events associated with the index hospitalization. Three independent raters rated the charts of these patients for precipitating events associated with the onset of psychosis. A precipitating stress was included as an item if at least two raters found it relevant in an individual case. The following categories of stress were identified: medical stresses, stress associated with loss or threatened loss of a supportive relationship, stress associated with role change demand, stress associated with marriage or parenting, and stress associated with vocational or financial problems. (For more details, see Table 1.) An inspection of Table 1 would indicate that

TABLE 1

Stressful Events Associated with the Onset of
Psychosis in Mid-Life

Category	Items
Medical stresses	Termination of therapeutic medication; use of provocative drugs (stimulants, hallucinogens, steroids); physical illness, surgery, disability; pregnancy or abortion; childbirth.
Stress associated with loss or threatened loss of a supportive relationship	Termination of professional therapeutic relationship; death of a family member; death of a close friend; loss of love relationship (non-marital) or threatened loss; recent move; change or threatened change in other close relationship (parent, sibling, adult son or daughter); severe illness in family member or close relationship.
Stress associated with role change demand	Concern over non-marital status; increased intimacy demand in love relationship; mid-life role change demand; mid-life role change in spouse; retirement.
Stress associated with marriage or parenting	Overt marital discord; marital divorce or separation; guilt over extra-marital affair; marital estrangement (without overt discord or separation); problem with phase-appropriate emancipation of children; other child rearing problem (i.e., limit setting); excessive intrusion in marriage by parent or in-law.
Stress associated with vocational or financial problems	Threatened or actual decrease in vocational or economic status; job loss; threatening increase in vocational status; actual or feared loss of financial support; legal problems.

the identified stressful events represent many normative stress points in mid-life. Table 2 shows the stressful events most frequently rated in our subjects. From an examination of these events, it appears that the stresses most commonly associated with the onset of psychosis in our group impeded the developmental goals of health maintenance, family solidarity, and vocational stability.

As a second approach to the life stresses in these patients, we used the subjective experience of psychotic patients as a window toward understanding the developmental impasse facing them. The follow-

TABLE 2

Ten Most Common Stressful Events Associated with the
Onset of Psychosis in Mid-Life

Events	Percent of Total Group
Physical illness, surgery, disability	24
Change or threatened change in other close relationship	21
Overt marital discord	18
Recent move	16
Actual or feared loss of financial support	14
Job loss	13
Severe illness in family member or close relationship	13
Intrusion in marriage by parents or in-laws	11
Discontinuation of therapeutic medication	11
Problem with phase-appropriate emancipation of children	11

ing two documents written by patients illustrate the developmental tasks confronting patients at the onset of their psychosis.

The first is an account illustrating an episode of psychosis associated with marital crisis. One week following the beginning of a six-week hospital stay, a 32-year-old married woman, at the request of the first author, agreed to write about her current marital difficulties. She apparently agreed to write the account to "have the whole experience behind me," and in that frame of mind she presented it. The immediate events leading up to hospitalization are alluded to in the document. Elizabeth was a very sensitive, though nonassertive, woman who was experiencing increasing conflict in her marriage of eight years. Her own father was an extremely critical and demanding man whose influence Elizabeth had hoped to escape by her marriage. Her husband, she increasingly perceived, was not the capable, protecting man she had hoped but was quite insecure and in need of support himself. His responses to her inadequacies were frequently thoughtless and abusive. He suggested, for instance, that she "go have some affairs" so that she could be a more satisfying sexual partner for him. She was, however, bound to the relationship by the same lack of confidence which made her relatively ineffective in it. In the context of this conflict she became psychotic, and she wrote the following document as a description of the onset of that experience:

It began at the first session of a class on the disciplining of children. My husband and I went together, and there were four other couples.

Earlier in the fall, I had told the leader about my marital problems and how worried I was because of what it might be doing to my children. As she talked, I began to think she had consulted other people about my husband and myself, even my parents and neighbors, and was using facts from my life to illustrate discipline situations. I was very happy that she had decided to help me, as it seemed to me. From things she said, I believed she had consulted our pediatrician. I thought of him as the kind of man I would have liked to have had as a father. I thought that he would be present at a social gathering scheduled for the Sunday after Valentine's Day, though I had no reason to suspect this. The group leader commented how important to a child's security and peace of mind was the care for his physical needs. I thought I had paid too much attention to my children's emotional needs forgetting the importance of their physical welfare. I thought Sandra, my daughter, might have a heart condition because I had pushed her too much. I thought both of the children might become deaf due to my failure to take them to the doctor in time. I felt guilty about smoking when I was pregnant with Ellen and when I nursed her. I thought that smoking was injuring my own health; sometimes I tried to stop, other times I wished I were dead, and smoked even the dirty cigarette butts lying around.

I believed that I was an "emotionally disturbed" person; I believed my husband was something or other, but I didn't know what except that it scared me to think he might break down and "do something." As she talked, the group leader's eyes had a twinkle. Later, when I began to think I had been hypnotized, I thought it had started that evening. Thoughts spun around in my head and everything, objects, sounds, events, took on special meaning for me. Childhood feelings began to come back, as symbols and bits from past conversations went through my head.

This account illustrates the kind of ideation related to striving for adult development that may occur in some psychotic episodes. Consider, for example, these passages:

I felt like I was putting the pieces of a puzzle together. I thought understanding myself better would help me with conflicts that I thought compelled to resolve; I wanted to grow up and feel the way a 32-year-old woman was supposed to . . . I felt as if I were love and hate with nothing in the middle, that everything was opposites, but that I was fighting myself so that the little girl of four and a half would grow up quickly and so that I could be a woman and a good mother to my children.

The timing of this psychotic illness is related to Elizabeth's perception that her marriage is in serious difficulty. She has endured years of abuse and disrespect which she has been unable to question; moreover, she blames herself for her husband's erratic, uncaring behavior. Intimidated throughout her early years by her own father, she now finds herself unable to manage that degree of healthy self-assertion as an adult which would have been required for the maintenance of her marriage. Her guilt and lack of competence in her role as wife and mother paralyze her, as does her fear that her husband will abandon her. Seemingly, it is this developmental impasse that ushers in the psychotic illness.

The next account illustrates the inner experiences of a man in the throes of vocational and marital stress. James was in his early 30s, married, with two children. He had recently changed assignments in his company and had a new boss who was distant and hard to approach. His previous boss had been open, helpful and supportive. In addition, James' new assignment had required that he learn some new technical procedures, and he felt he might have difficulty with these new tasks. He felt, therefore, that his job might be in jeopardy. He was afraid he might get fired and be unable to support his family. His sexual drive had declined during this period of concern over his job, and his wife was complaining about his lack of sexual interest. During long commutes to work he began to think that he should have a homosexual experience. He was frightened by such fantasies yet felt that he should force himself to do it so that he could overcome his fear of trying new things. Three months prior to admission for acute psychosis, he had a casual homosexual encounter and recorded his thoughts and feelings in the weeks that followed.

When two people enter into marriage they bring themselves. But the wife is destined to occupy an unusual position, she must assume the husband's name. If the roles were reversed, the husband would occupy an unequal position. Instead, when they marry they should assume a new name, any name. Perhaps that is what is needed to break with tradition. We have been taught that sex is something special, that it must be protected and given out only under the most restricted circumstances. If we give it under any other circumstances, it is bad. Yet we constantly have these physical desires which we must suppress with our minds. We put our physical and mental beings in constant conflict with each other, and there is no peace within us. Worse than that, by using our energies to combat each other, we keep ourselves from growing, from becoming fully aware. Why would we build a wall within us that keeps us in constant conflict with ourselves? Suddenly I am very fearful; I am fearful that I will discover something that I cannot comprehend. I am on a planet, flying through space which has been set on course many years ago by a great power. I am going to have to make contact with those directing the flight. I must do something drastic before I am able to recognize them with my senses. Eventually I will outgrow them. Should I wait until I outgrow them before I risk being discovered or would my growth stop if I did not make the effort? I know I want to keep growing. Anger is one of our senses. We must not suppress it. It occurs to me that anger causes quarrels. Why must children fight and hit each other? Let us learn to make our friendships both mental and physical. In the whole United States I don't think there is one happy family. Is there any family that does not quarrel? We have been directed to concentrate our energies on fighting one another. What a joy life would be if we were able to give to each other freely. My mind is growing by leaps and bounds. How will it affect my life? Perhaps I should slow down. The more I think, the more I stimulate more thoughts. I must take a rest.

James grew up in a family where he and his father had little interaction. He once commented that his father said that James was lucky just to have a roof over his head. James was severely limited by his inability to share his inner life, his deepest concerns with others, even his wife. Encountering doubts and questions in his work and his marriage, he had limited autonomous resources to sustain him. He sought intimacy and understanding in a casual homosexual experience but was inevitably deeply disappointed. The ensuing guilt only added to his private burden. In this context, he developed an acute psychosis.

As noted by Dr. Lidz in Chapter 2 of this volume, the making of a marriage obviously builds upon the relatively successful transition from adolescence to young adulthood. Psychosis occurring in marriage usually indicates that this process has been impaired. Needs unmet in the primary family become the determinants of object choice, and usually these needs obscure the true person of the potential spouse and cause one to seize upon superficial characteristics. Here again relationship-making is impaired by the urgency of the inner need which makes accurate, reality-based, protracted scrutiny of a potential spouse difficult. Further, in a growing marriage, the capacity to provide, rather than be provided for, gets called upon. Thus, marriage severely tests the capacity for internal maintenance of self-esteem at times when the environment fails to gratify. In the best of relationships, adult intimacy appears to actually foster the growth of autonomy and the ability to bear loneliness or the relative absence of object gratification. These capacities are crucial for growth in later years.

As illustrated in the accounts of these patients, growth strivings may be evident in the subjective experience of the psychotic individual. This phenomenon has been noted by a number of clinicians, perhaps beginning with Mayer-Gross who wrote a monograph on the course of the acute psychoses (Mayer-Gross, 1920). One of the outcomes he delineated was that associated with actual developmental progress. Anton Boisen, a chaplain at a hospital in Illinois, wrote a series of papers and two books dealing with the identification of some psychoses as problem-solving experiences (Boisen, 1952, 1960). Harry Stack Sullivan (1962) felt that the single most critical factor in prognosis was the individual's perception of this growth impasse and his self-assessment of his ability to overcome the impasse.

But in what sense can psychoses be called impasses in growth and what is the therapist's proper response? I think there is some confusion on this point and the clinician can be easily misled. In acute psychotic states some individuals experience a coalescence of meaning, a kind of epiphany which may appeal to the romantic side of some therapists. The psychedelic drugs have taught us—if one did not already know from experience—that the experience of meaning bears no relationship to ultimate empirical facts (Bowers and Freedman, 1966). Some clinicians may be tempted to collude with the acutely psychotic patient in the search for psychological meaning, as if this state were a once in a lifetime opportunity. This temptation, in our opinion, should be resisted. This opinion does not mean that the growth strivings manifest in acute psychotic experience are meaningless. Such impulses may be regarded (and explained to patient) as an expression of hope, a manifestation of a positive life at work within the individual. They bear the same relationship to growth as the creative idea to a finished work or the dream of a reformer like Martin Luther King to the achievement of desegregation in fact (Bowers, 1971).

In recent years, a number of treatments have been promulgated under the assumption that the psychotic state itself is a special opportunity for psychological growth. These programs are illustrated in the writings of Ronald Laing and in the more systematic research conducted under the leadership of Loren Mosher at Soteria House in California. It does seem possible for selected patients to recover from their psychoses in three to six months without medication in an environment which permits, even encourages, patients to work with the content of their psychotic experiences. This option is really not a viable alternative in most treatment settings, however. Most experienced therapists feel that genuine psychological work cannot be undertaken while the patient is psychotic. True growth is arduous and needs to be pursued with one's feet on the ground.

The first task for therapist and patient in these conditions is the establishment of a therapeutic alliance. There may be unique difficulties in the establishment of a working relationship with a patient who has been psychotic and who continues to be vulnerable to psychotic episodes. Most of these individuals will need antipsychotic medication and they must be willing to give up aspects of psychotic experience which may be exhilarating and gratifying.

Once appropriate medication with minimum side effects has been negotiated, attention can be directed to the developmental tasks confronting the patient. Since many of the developmental issues in this group center on the family, the therapist must be prepared to include the spouse regularly or intermittently in the treatment process. In our experience, it is difficult but not impossible for a marriage to survive if one member becomes psychotic. It becomes clear relatively soon in the therapy whether or not the union is viable. If separation or divorce ensues, the therapist must be prepared to support the patient through this difficult transition. In our experience, the vulnerability of individual patients to recurrent psychotic episodes varies considerably. In a successful treatment, the patient ultimately assumes the responsibility for periodic or continuous use of medication if necessary to avoid relapse. Use of medication may continue even after regular psychotherapeutic sessions have ceased. The therapist remains indefinitely as a source of support and guidance during crisis periods.

In summary, this analysis suggests that the normative stresses of adult development are precisely those issues which are problematic for individuals who become psychotic in mid-life. The therapist is usually left to help these individuals wrestle with these growth tasks no matter what etiological role they play. Individuals who become psychotic at this point in life usually have some interpersonal accomplishments to build upon so that therapeutic efforts may be particularly rewarding.

REFERENCES

BOISEN, A.: *The Exploration of the Inner World.* New York: Harper & Row, 1952.

BOISEN, A.: *Out of the Depths.* New York: Harper & Row, 1960.

BOWERS, M. B., JR.: Psychosis and human growth. *The Human Context,* 1971, 3:134-145.

BOWERS, M. B., JR.: *Retreat from Sanity: The Structure of Emerging Psychosis.* New York: Human Sciences Press, 1974.

BOWERS, M. B., JR.: Clinical components of psychotic disorders: Their relationship to treatment. *Schizophrenia Bulletin,* 1977, 3:600-607.

BOWERS, M. B., JR. & FREEDMAN, D. X.: Psychedelic experiences in acute psychoses. *Archives of General Psychiatry,* 1966, 15, 240-246.

MAYER-GROSS, W.: Uber die stellungnahme zur abgelaufenen akuten psychose. *Zeitschrift für die Neurologie und Psychiatrie,* 1920, 60:160-212.

PHILLIPS, L.: Case history data and prognosis in schizophrenia. *Journal of Nervous and Mental Disease,* 1953, 117:515-525.

SULLIVAN, H.: *Schizophrenia as a Human Process.* New York: W. W. Norton and Co., 1962.

SPITZER, R., ENDICOTT, J., & ROBINS, E.: Research diagnostic criteria: Rationale and reliability. Paper presented at the American Psychiatric Association, Toronto, Canada, 1977.

Chapter 6

Changing Roles for Women at Mid-Life

Malkah Tolpin Notman

Until quite recently, studies investigating adult development have stressed the significance of loss and decline and have regarded this phase within the life cycle as a relatively static period between adolescence and old age. Within the past decade, however, the emphasis has changed towards a perception of the middle years as a time of development and growth rather than one where the major dynamic is toward aging and death (Gould, 1972; Barnett and Baruch, 1978; Neugarten, 1975). Although recent research has stressed opportunities and change, much of this may be designed to reassure the writer as well as the reader, since aging continues to be dreaded in a culture which emphasizes youth. It is apparent that women at mid-life, for instance, have anticipated with dread the onset of menopause and view it as termination, rather than change. The major focus of this paper will be on change and adaptation rather than loss and decline. Within this context, the chapter will address the changing roles of women at mid-life.

DEFINITIONS OF MIDDLE AGE

A definition of middle age has not been easy to attain. Levinson, Darrow, Klein, Levinson and McKee (1978) have argued for an age-related definition, based on the concept that fairly universal stages take place at certain ages or within age ranges. This point of view has been challenged by Neugarten (1975), who questions whether a view of life applicable to the developmental stages of infancy and childhood is equally applicable to adult life. Moreover, it would appear that using chronological age as a basis for developmental stages does not adequately account for individual differences and environmental events. Neugarten (1968), for example, in a study of "100 well-placed men and women" in middle age observed that chronological age was a less important marker for people in middle age than it was for the young or elderly. The women, but not the men, in this group defined their age status in terms of timing of events within the family cycle. For married women, middle age was closely tied to the launching of children into the adult world, and even unmarried career women often discussed middle age in terms of the family they might have had. This family-based definition is important, although it may be shifting in the context of current social changes, with work and careers occupying a greater role for women than they did at the time of Neugarten's study. However, this observation points to an important issue; most studies of development and the concepts which have been derived from these studies have been based on work with men and with models appropriate to male development. Women's development, recognized as different, has been conceptualized as deviant from the primary male normative pattern (Barnett and Baruch, 1978; Gilligan and Notman, 1978). Male subjects have been used for most studies until quite recently, and life cycle theorists have implicitly adopted the male pattern as the developmental norm, generally failing to recognize the extent to which this has been so and the fashion in which this colors accepted ideas about women.

Changing this pattern of research involves an alteration in conceptualization in which the lives of women would become the primary subject for observation. Views about women would no longer be derived from modification of ideas about men. Current work has begun to approach this to some extent (Barnett and Baruch, 1978), but a full developmental psychology of women does not yet exist.

One further consequence of the reliance on male patterns has been the acceptance of a linear progression of development in which an individual is seen as passing through a definite series of stages. Here, too, the apropriateness of this model, which is generally accepted for children, may be questioned for adults. Barnett and Baruch (1978), for example, point out that resolution of issues of identity and autonomy may take place only partially in early adult years to be replaced by the developmental experiences of motherhood and then resumed when children are grown. Women may occupy different role patterns at different times, with different combinations of children, work and marriage. The stage of family development in relation to age of children and their presence or absence in the family is also an important determinant of a woman's own life stages. Gilligan and Notman (1978) also discuss the differences in sequence of development for men and women, where for women "autonomy" and "identity" are not followed by "intimacy" as outlined in the Eriksonian sequence but can be thought of as part of a more simultaneous development. This is consistent with the data showing that women are more embedded in social interaction and personal relationships than men.

Freud (1933) tried to fit women into his masculine conception. He saw them as envying that which they missed, and only later came to recognize the strength and persistence of women's pre-oedipal attachments to mother as a developmental difference. However, he considered this difference responsible for what he perceived as the woman's developmental failure. Deprived of the impetus for a clear-cut Oedipal resolution which was in his thinking provided for boys by castration anxiety, women's supergo was consequently compromised. As Freud described this difference, a woman's superego is "never so inexorable, impersonal, and so independent of its emotional origins as we require it to be in men." He concluded, echoing, he said, critics of every epoch, "that women have less sense of justice than men, that they are more often influenced in their judgments by feelings of affection and hostility, and by general concern for others" (Freud, 1933) .

Similarly, Kohlberg (1964) , in his theory of moral development, perceived the end goal of moral development as a commitment to an abstract sense of principle. Women reached their abstract goal more infrequently than men because of their ties to other people, which in Freud's terms was a corruption of a sense of justice, and in Kohlberg's terms is a failure to develop. For boys and men, separation and individuation, independence and the capacity for aggressive activity are critically tied to the development of masculinity since separation from one's mother is critical to the development of masculine identity. For girls and women, by contrast, issues of femininity of feminine identity do not require the same separation. Girls will tend to have problems with separation and individuation whereas boys' difficulties will have more to do with intimacy and attachment. The greater involvement in personal relationships which characterizes women's lives in comparison to men's becomes not only a descriptive difference but is often perceived as a developmental liability, although an important component of femininity. Since the milestones of childhood and adolescent development are defined in terms of autonomy and separation, women's failure to achieve these, such as the failure to separate, measured in the same terms, is seen as a failure to develop rather than a different direction of development (Gilligan and Notman, 1978) .

If separation and autonomy, which have been essentially masculine goals, are seen as the end point of development, then the kind of relatedness which women maintain is seen as a reflection of inadequate maturity. This "relatedness" is not the same as "dependency," which concerns the need fulfilling character of relationships, with no choice nor separateness. "Relatedness" is a conception of one's life as closely associated with fulfillment via others and bound up with the welfare of others (Erikson, 1963; Miller, 1976) .

Separation-individuation becomes an important mid-life issue because of the many separations which must be managed. These experiences are better conceptualized as separations rather than as

losses. Women are vulnerable to separation since they define themselves strongly and consistently in terms of their relationships with
others and seem sensitive to and dependent on the opinions of
others. This is part of the legacy of feminine development. In
adolescence, according to Erikson (1963), the developmental task
is the emergence of identity and autonomy. As we have seen, the
resolution of the tasks of adolescence is somewhat different for women, since not only does intimacy accompany identity, given sufficient separation and individuation in early life, but women's identity is not as autonomously defined as that of men. They have
generally been considered through the identity of others—their parents, husbands and children.

From the preceding comments, it seems apparent that the linear
stages of adult development may not be so helpful for a meaningful
concept of women's mid-life. What then constitutes adult development for women? What is an appropriate conception or definition
of mid-life?

Having criticized a definition based on age, or the achievement
of uniformly defined "stages," one must look to another approach.
Neugarten (1968) stresses the following characteristics of middle
age: a heightened sensitivity to one's position within a complex social environment, and the theme of reassessment of the self. The
difference in the time perspective and recognition of the finiteness of
time are frequently cited themes of mid-life. Time left to live becomes an important concern rather than the infinite sense of time
of youth.

It is important to also take into account the social definition of
a particular life stage. Giele (1977) observes that as a country
modernizes, for example, it tends to lengthen childhood and youth
and refines stages into more precise time periods with special developmental tasks expected for more differentiated and separated
age groups. She draws a parallel between this development in relation to stages of youth and early adulthood and the current elabora-
tion of stages of middle adulthood and offers the actual extension
of the total life span in recent years as one explanation. Changes in
patterns of work and family life have led to smaller families and a
longer post-parental period. These factors also help identify the

middle years as a distinct phase of life. Giele also emphasizes that the new concepts of adulthood involve a change in definition of sex roles as well as age roles. The very ideology of mid-life development implies growth of the personality to encompass some characteristics that had stereotypically in the past been assigned to the opposite sex.

Levinson et al.'s (1978) conceptualization of life stages observed in their studies of men places central importance on the role of work in establishing oneself in the world. Although the importance of family relationships for the adult man is acknowledged, they are not the organizing theme of his life. In his own development, separation from his family of origin is placed more centrally than the birth of his first child.

For women, as we have seen, the life course is somewhat different. We have referred to women's tendency to define themselves in terms of others and to conceptualize their middle age in relation to their families. There are two important components of this definition: one is the limitation on women's reproductive lives imposed by the biological timetable, and the other is the close association of a woman's concept of her life stage with the phase of family development.

There has been a tendency to describe women's lives as more strongly determined by biological forces than men's. For example, women have been seen as more vulnerable to hormonal influences and "natural" forces and therefore less able to maintain control of their lives (Ortner, 1974). While one might question the "raging hormone" theory, in which a woman's state of mind is seen as being under the influence of her hormonal status, as expressing prejudice unsupported by data, certainly biology and, in particular, fertility have determined the phases of development for women more critically than for men. Unfortunately, these factors become stereotyped as being inevitably the central determinants. The biological clock does constitute a constant reminder and framework for life, compellingly limiting the options for childbearing. For men, there is no correspondingly clear limit.

As previously discussed, an important and central characteristic of middle age is awareness of the finiteness of time. Thus, for women this awareness of their middle age is closely related to the possibility of choice about having children. This possibility ends at menopause. Although, in adolescence, both boys and girls reach sexual and reproductive maturity with dramatic endocrine and physical changes, the adult man does not experience any further biological event in which his life options are as definitely changed by the functioning of his body as the cessation of the menses is for women. However, although the hormonal and physical changes mark major periods of a woman's life, the characteristics and experiences of these periods may be less related to the actual biological change than has been assumed. The separation of the biological and social life cycles has also meant that the time of actual childbearing corresponds less to the beginning and end of fertility than in the past.

We thus return to the question of an appropriate conception of mid-life. Age alone does not provide this. We have seen that considerations involving children and their lives are important for women. Neugarten (1978) defined middle age as beginning with "launching" one's children into the world. Alice Rossi (1968) also considers a definition related to children (i.e., with the end of parenting at the marriage of children). However, there has been an increasing spread in the age at which the first child is born because of women's variable phasing of career and family, with many more women deciding to have children later, thus increasing the numbers of older primiparas. The increase in adolescent pregnancies and young mothers pushes the age range at one end and the number of remarriages and second families also pushes it at the other. So starting parenthood corresponds less and less to a fixed chronological age of the mother, and the developmental stages of the children occur at varying periods in her own life and family development. The ages of one's children often determine with whom one associates, and critical family events such as the exit of the first or last child which are important in defining life stages occur at different points in the chronological, personal or professional life of an individual woman.

A clinical syndrome occurring for some women in their early 30s presents a paradoxial aspect of a mid-life crisis, one which takes place at the beginning rather than the end of childbearing. This can be labeled the "age 30 crisis." It is also a point at which a woman may come for psychotherapy. At about the age of 30, many women feel they will no longer have an uncomplicated choice about childbearing. Gynecological opinions, based on past experiences with "elderly primiparas," support the view that a woman should have her first child by age 30, and this is often stated without much regard for the individual woman's maturity or readiness for childbearing. This is no longer universally subscribed to (Friedman, 1978), but nevertheless remains in the popular culture and is still supported by some obstetricians.

Some people have their own special age—the magic period of transition is somewhat different, perhaps 35 or 40. But by and large 30 has been the important birthday which marks the transition from youth. Even those women who are not interested in having children feel aware of that choice as a decision to be made as they approach 30. This may involve reworking an earlier decision, sometimes unconsciously. If they feel the possibility of their having children is remote, because they are unmarried or because they are far from resolving their ambivalence, there may be depression and mourning for a part of themselves and for potential life plans that will never be realized. Other women feel anxiety that time is slipping away, and concerns which once seemed remote and postponable, such as problems in relationships, suddenly become urgent. Some women come for help at this time for symptoms of depression or anxiety without really being aware of the reasons. A birthday, a loss of a relationship, a move in a career direction which is interpreted as an increased commitment to a childless state may bring about a depression. The awareness of the finiteness of time to carry out one's fantasies and wishes which has been repeatedly pointed to as characterizing mid-life is thus also connected with the possibility of choosing or being able to have children before the end of the childbearing period. It is a psychological mid-life issue which may be unrelated to the actual menopause, although it does perhaps involve contemplation of this approaching. Obviously, not all women want children; childbearing and parenting are often stressful. However, confrontation with choices is important and forms a part of every woman's self-concept and self-awareness. Developmental stages for women are thus produced by an interweaving of those experiences related to childbirth, parenting and family development, with those experiences relating to the establishment of separations and autonomy, personal identity, intellectual growth and relationship to work.

The loss of youth itself is also more critical for women than men. Sontag (1972) has described the double standard of aging which penalizes women more than men. Since the reproductive timetable is less rigid for a man, his reaching his thirtieth birthday does not have the same impact as for a woman, both because of the social acceptability of increasing age and the lack of a specific restriction of options for having a family as he get older.

Freud ascribed the psychological differences between men and women as they enter mid-life to differences in their nature. While making allowances for individual differences, he writes (Freud, 1933) that: "A man of about thirty strikes us as a youthful, somewhat uniformed individual, whom we expect to make a powerful use of the possibilities for development opened up to him by analysis. A woman of the same age, however, often frightens us by her physical rigidity and unchangeability" (p. 135). As Freud saw it, a man's development in work and other areas in his life was felt to be still open. A woman at 30 was already entrenched in her role, and other possibilities for growth and development were not apparent, as if the difficult development to femininity had exhausted the possibilities for further growth of the person concerned.

A clinical example illustrates one aspect of the problem:

> Ms B., a young psychologist, became depressed when given a responsible position, in effect, in charge of a special ward, which she had previously wanted very much. She was angry at the physicians who did not spend enough time there and who asked her to assume more responsibility and authority and involved her in the planning for the unit. This new position moved her up the career ladder, a move she had also previously thought she wanted. She was puzzled about her depressive reaction and sought consultation.

Recently she had ended a five-year relationship with a man which had been close and warm, although not entirely satisfactory. He was clearly never going to marry and she had been disappointed and angry that the relationship was not "getting anywhere," although at the same time she expressed ambivalence about marriage.

Her family background was a troubled one. Her relationships with her parents were difficult. Her father had been ill and disabled, always emotionally absent, and had died when she was in high school. Her mother, with whom she often had clashed, had been depressed and then alcoholic. One brother had dropped out of school, another younger brother was still at home, at loose ends. One sister had recurrent marital problems and was in the process of divorce. She herself had always had been ambivalent about having children because of her poor relationship with her mother and the constant turmoil in the family. She had been the family caretaker, an adaptation which had lead her into psychology. There, her intelligence and resourcefulness had resulted in her success and promotion. She had thought that was her goal. Although she had felt convinced that she did not want children, with the disruption of the relationship with the man, it seemed less likely that she would ever permit herself the opportunity to have children. At the time of her thirtieth birthday, she found herself mourning the possibility she felt she was losing. The responsibilities of the job seemed to make concrete that she was taking a further step away from the alternate way of life which would involve marriage and family.

Among young professional women, reaching 30 also may precipitate a reexamination of life plans. Sometimes an "inadvertent pregnancy" results, expressing the unconscious or partially conscious wish for a child. After the disorganization and disruption of plans are settled, this may be accepted or even welcomed, since it may provide a resolution of the conflict which might have been difficult to arrive at consciously. If carrying through the pregnancy produces severe stress, the availability of abortion offers an opportunity to interrupt it and continue with plans for work or other directions but it precipitates into consciousness one aspect of the conflict.

MENOPAUSE

Turning to a closer examination of actual middle age for women brings us to a consideration of the menopause. Menopause has been stereotyped as providing the dominant factor in women's mid-life phase. In clinical considerations of patients who present with depression or other symptomatology, there has been a tendency to focus automatically on the menstrual history, as if it will explain the symptomatology of the patient. Actually, the relationships are not all that inevitable or clear (McKinley and Jefferys, 1974; McKinley and McKinley, 1973; Neugarten and Kraines, 1965; and Notman, 1976). Research in this area has been relatively sparse and uneven. It has been criticized methodologically for failure to develop consistent definitions and for sloppiness of sampling and approach.

Many misconceptions have existed about the nature and extent of menopausal symptoms. McKinley and McKinley (1973), in a review of the menopause literature, and Parlee (1976) point to the lack of attention to menopause in the medical literature and are critical of the research which does exist. They cite methodological problems such as the failure to develop consistent objective definitions of menopause and of menopausal symptomatology, the use of retrospective data, case histories, clinical impressions and the analysis of data obtained from selected samples of women who are under the care of gynecologists and psychiatrists. Those studies they considered more reliable show that psychosomatic and psychological complaints were not reported more frequently by so-called "menopausal" than by younger women (Neugarten, Wood, Kraines and Loomis, 1968). Some have seen the paucity of good research about a phenomenon which has been in existence for a very long time as a reflection of the lack of interest of male researchers in women's lives and problems. In a review of endocrinological data, Perlmutter (1978) suggests that there are multiple disorders that have been ascribed to the changing hormonal balance and are equated with menopause. In reality, not all of the changes that are noted are due to hormonal imbalances; some are the consequences of aging and others have a basis in psychological factors and life patterns.

Menopause is defined as the cessation of the menses for one year, and thus is a diagnosis which is made retrospectively. A more appropriate term for this period would be the perimenopausal years. During this time there is a gradual diminution of ovarian function and a gradual change in endocrine status (Perlmutter, 1977). Age of menopause varies from the late 30s to middle or even late 50s. This variation supports the tendency to assign a variety of symptoms occurring in these years to a woman's menopausal status. In a study of age at menopause, McKinley, Jefferys and Thompson (1972) found that the median age of menopause in industrial societies is about 50 years of age. There is no firm evidence that this age has increased, at least in the last century, nor any indication of a close relationship between the age at menopause and the age at menarche or socioeconomic status. "There is some evidence that marital status and parity are related to the age at menopause, independently of each other" (p. 113).

The lack of estrogen due to diminished ovarian production causes the increased production of stimulating hormones from the hypothalamus and pituitary, which in some unknown way affect the heat-regulating mechanism of the body. The hot flashes and sweats may not be particularly visible to an outsider but may be an acute source of embarrassment to an individual woman, who can be reassured to learn that they are not detected by others.

What is the symptomatology directly attributable to the menopause? Vasomotor instability, manifested as hot flashes, flushes, episodes of perspiration or attacks, is one of the consistent symptoms accompanying menopause (McKinley and Jefferys, 1974; Reynolds, 1962). This is present in up to 75 percent of women who report some degree of symptomatology. McKinley and Jefferys (1974), in a review of symptoms of women aged 45 to 54 in the London area, found that "hot flushes and night sweats are clearly associated with the onset of a natural menopause and that they occur in a majority of women." The other symptoms investigated, namely, "headaches, dizzy spells, palpitations, sleeplessness, depressions, and weight increase, showed no direct relationship to the menopause but tended to occur together." The length of time a woman experiences the hot flashes is variable. They may originate several years before actual menopause, and can be considered a sign of waning estrogen levels, reaching a peak at about the time of the actual cessation of the menses and persisting as long as five years (Perlmutter, 1977). It should be noted, however, that etiology of the hot flashes remains unclear and appears to be related to hormonal imbalance between the hypothalamus, pituitary, and ovary rather than simple estrogen deficit (Reynolds, 1962).

The vasomotor instability is of varying severity and duration and is also experienced in widely different ways. Some women are distressed at their lack of control over their bodies which evokes anxieties about regression and control of other somatic functions. For others, the potential visibility of the flush is most prominent. Some women are concerned about revealing their menopause or sexual states. Since the flushes are confined to the upper part of the body, similar to the blush area (Barnett and Baruch, 1978), one might speculate about the emotional issues of shame as well as other feelings which might be potentially associated with the symptoms.

Psychological factors such as anger, anxiety, and excitement are considered important in precipitating flushes in susceptible women, as are activities giving rise to excess heat production or retention, such as a warm environment, muscular work, and eating hot food (Reynolds, 1962). However, the symptoms may arise without any clear psychological or heat-stimulating mechanism.

Other symptoms which have been attributed to the menopause have included a wide variety of complaints. These really do not seem to be directly attributable to the actual menopause. Insomnia, irritability, depression, diminished sexual interest, headaches, dizzy spells, and palpitations have been considered part of the menopausal period by some but they do not occur consistently and in fact may be depressive symptoms or indications of anxiety (Bart and Grossman, 1978; McKinlay and Jefferys, 1974). For instance, in Neugarten's studies (Neugarten and Datan, 1974; Neugarten and Kraines, 1965) menopausal status is not associated with measurable anxiety.

Many other mid-life changes have been attributed to menopause and many symptoms thought to be menopausal have been attributed to estrogen deficiency or other hormonal effects. Neugarten and Kraines (1965) studied 100 women aged 43 to 53 using menstrual histories as an index of menopausal status. They found climacteric (menopausal) status to be unrelated to a wide array of personality measures. They also found very few significant relationships between the severity of any somatic and psychosomatic symptoms and these personality variables. Bart and Grossman (1978) found that menopausal status was not a contributing factor in self-evaluations of middle-aged women. They also found, as one might expect, that women who had low self-esteem and low levels of life satisfaction were more likely to have difficulties with menopause. These and other data indicate that women's reactions to important transition points in their lives, such as menarche and pregnancy, are consistent with their reactions to menopause. Thus, one can consider menopause as one of the important experiences for women that is best understood in the context of their entire lives, and their particular experiences and adaptive responses.

For many years, menopause was considered a deficiency disease due to the lowered estrogen levels. Although the ovaries do diminish estrogen production and the menstrual cycles cease, Perlmutter (1978) cites a number of conditions also associated with low estrogen levels, such as anorexia nervosa, and, on occasion, abrupt surgical menopause, where there are no hot flashes. However, when lowered estrogen levels occur because of menopause, the condition is often viewed as a deficiency with the emphasis on loss rather than the possibility of progression into the next stage of life where a woman is protected from pregnancy and can turn to other activities. Another assumption implicit in the deficiency disease model is that the normal state for women is one of reproductive activity. One might instead consider this phase of a woman's life (i.e. menopause) as another phase within a series of normal developmental stages. For the prepubertal girl, low estrogen levels are normal, as they are for the post-menopausal woman. There are indeed changes in skin, mucosa, possible muscle tone, which are attributed to post-menopausal estrogen diminution. However, these are also part of the aging process. In any event, high estrogen secretion in a 60-year-old woman is not considered normal but an indication of disease.

The idea that reproductive potential and the core of feminine normality are the same is reflected in early psychoanalytic writing on the subject. Menopause was conceptualized by psychoanalytic theoreticians largely in terms of loss. Helene Deutsch (1946) spoke of a "narcissistic mortification" that is difficult to overcome and suggested that the woman "loses all she received during puberty." She also noted that "mastery of the psychologic reactions to the organic decline is one of the most difficult tasks of a woman's life." Deutsch saw it as a narcissistic blow which is so real that psychotherapy could not really offer much to make up for it. She saw the post-menopausal increase in the activity of women and in their interest in work, which has been well-known clinically as a "struggle to preserve femininity," which in turn was tied with sexual attractiveness and reproductive possibilities. It was as if these women were saying, "If I cannot have any more children, I must look for something else." Deutsch felt that the focus on work was compensatory for the loss of sexuality and femininity, and did not perceive it as an expression of primary interests.

Benedek (1950) believed menopause was a time of difficulty and of complex and demanding personal and social tasks for women. They must adapt to grown and more independent children, changing sexual relations with husbands, and changing responses to life. She believed not all women experienced it as similarly stressful, but she saw the problem as greater for women who had not borne children. Benedek believed the disturbance would be greater in women who were less "feminine" and had not had gratification from motherliness. She did feel the energy released by no longer being involved in reproductive tasks gave women with flexible egos impetus for learning and socialization. Benedek and most others of that period saw the mother as primarily involved with children and did not consider fathers or family dynamics fully in relation to child rearing or in relation to responses of women to menopause.

Benedek and Deutsch held that a woman's reaction to menopause was similar to her reaction to puberty and pregnancy. However, early writers stressed the aspect of loss rather than adaptation to change. The former view reflects the concept of feminine identity as strongly related to reproduction. When active childbearing ends, an important source of a woman's self-esteem is gone and she must mourn the outcome. Although for many individuals this may be true, this view does not allow for a concept of mid-life development in which one may progress to a developmental stage which is normal for a later period of life.

Sexual interest and responsiveness do not diminish at mid-life for women. Many women report increased sexual satisfaction as they are freed from anxiety about pregnancy. Although changes in patterns of response occur with age, particularly for men, Masters and Johnson (1966) document the maintenance of full sexual activity in middle-aged individuals and they stress the idea that the inevitable diminution of sexual function with age is a myth.

Benedek and Deutsch both agreed that reactions to menopause are similar to reactions to other important milestones in feminine development. They and other psychoanalysts predicted that women who were childless would be most likely to have difficulties when the childbearing period ends. Other past experiences were expected to resurface at menopause, for example, guilt or regret for a previous abortion. However, clinical and research data do not support this view. Women who experience the most distress at the time of menopause are those who have relied most on their childbearing role as a source of self-esteem, status, and importance in society. Data by Bart and Grossman (1978) and Neugarten and Kraines (1965), for example, indicate that women who have had children, have "high motherliness" scores on self-report scales, and have invested heavily in their childbearing and rearing, are more likely to experience depression. Women who have not had children do not necessarily have more difficulties at menopause. Many of them have had to come to terms with their childlessness earlier than the biological menopause and have found alternative ways to organize their lives. The menopause then represents a less critical event. To some extent, childlessness may represent underlying ambivalence about motherhood, which is more acceptable in contemporary society than earlier and can also be better implemented with effective contraception and abortion.

Depression has long been associated with menopause, but appears to be more clearly associated with psychosocial variables than with endocrine changes (Osopky and Seidenberg, 1970; Winokur, 1973) and is not inevitable. In an exhaustive review of the literature concerning the relationship of depression with female endocrine status, Weissman and Klerman (1977) conclude that because of poor methodology the relationship between endocrine status and clinical status remains questionable. They also suggest that the effect of menopause on increasing a woman's vulnerability to depression may be minimal. Other authors agree (Osopky and Seidenberg, 1970; Winokur, 1973) and cite the lack of studies which utilize modern endocrinological methods to investigate the relationship between depression and endocrine status. Based on the available research literature, mid-life does not appear to be the period of time in which women are most vulnerable to depression.

Social class represents another important variable to consider when investigating women's responses to menopause. For example, middle- and upper-class women when compared to lower-class women find the cessation of childbearing more liberating because more alternatives are available to them, and they are less anxious about menopause (Neugarten, 1968). Bart and Grossman (1978) suggest the following variables as relevant factors in determining women's response to menopause: social-economic status, attitude toward child rearing and mothering, and available alternatives. A woman who has given all her life to her children and feels useless when they are gone is more likely to feel depressed.

Anxiety about menopause is considerable among women but may be greater in the anticipation than in the actual experience. Neugarten (1968) found in her study of middle-class women that younger women anticipating menopause were more concerned than women who were actually menopausal. Post-menopausal women generally took a more positive view than pre-menopausal women and a higher proportion of them agreed that menopause creates no major discontinuity in life and that, except for the underlying biological changes, women have a considerable degree of control over their symptoms and need not inevitably have difficulties. Cross-cultural studies indicate that in those cultures where there is improved status at middle age and a clear role for the middle-aged woman, there are greater feelings of well-being at mid-life (Bart and Grossman, 1978). In our society, women whose lives have not been child-centered and for whom their marital ties remain or women whose children remain close and gratifying have an easier time at middle age and menopause.

Family experiences are important in determining the outcome of this period (Zilbach, 1975). The mid-life transition for men, often the husbands of menopausal women, also brings new stresses (Notman, 1977). This period for men is often accompanied by sexual problems, sometimes leading to affairs, marital disruption and the abandonment of their wives. Adolescent children may be sexually and aggressively provocative, challenging or disappointing. Here, too, there are important class differences in the readiness to have affairs and the availability of divorce. As noted by Dr. Gould in Chapter 7 of this volume, the increasing work opportunities for women have probably stimulated more women who are dissatisfied with their marriage to seek divorce than in the past.

SEPARATION

The adaptation to separations is an important developmental task at mid-life. The ability to separate from children as they grow and depart from home is only one of the separations to master. Here, too, however, is the implied element of loss. The family balance changes with the departure of the first child, and some women feel a conscious or unconscious impulse to replace the balance by having another child (Zilbach, 1975). On the other hand, some women experience this period as providing additional opportunities to pursue personal, educational and occupational interests. It would appear that women in the latter group do not perceive separation from children solely as a loss but as an opportunity for adding something to their lives. The "empty nest syndrome" does not appear to be a universal event. In fact, some families experience stress when adult children return home for awhile to refill the empty nest (Foote, 1978). This can create conflict for the woman who finds herself unable to decide whether to be a mother in the old sense and provide for everyone or attempt to redefine the role functions of the family as an adult community where she is free to pursue more of her own directions and needs.

It is important to note, however, that as children grow up there is less physical contact with them and if sexual interactions with husbands or others are waning, a total diminution of physical contact can occur. In this culture, individuals rarely touch each other, men even less than women. A woman may thus be left with a marked absence of occasions for physical closeness and warmth. If so, women who find themselves with a marked absence of physical contact may experience considerable difficulty adapting to separations.*

An important determinant of the capacity to deal with separations is the successful resolution of previous experiences with separation (Zilbach, 1975). If earlier separations are unresolved, separations from children or loss of one's husband may be particularly difficult. The child who leaves home may stir up unconscious memories of the previous loss of a parent, sibling, or other important person. The successful separation of the adolescent or young adult from his or her family may be unconsciously prevented by the parent who never worked through her/his own earlier losses.

Illness and death of elderly parents of people in mid-life precipitate the necessity to cope with separation and role changes. The illness or death of a parent can bring into sharp focus the awareness that this middle-aged person is now the dominant generation. This revives old memories and identifications, and may lead to anxiety as well as depression. The knowledge that one is the generation in power and control can be perceived in positive terms as well but is often accompanied by a sense of its impermanence (Gould, 1972; Neugarten, 1968).

Adolescence and mid-life have often been compared. Both are life transitions which specifically depend on a redefinition of the relationship between oneself and others and therefore these transitions

---

* I am indebted for this observation to Dr. Beatrice Whiting, who feels that the need for contact is one of the universal human needs and she points to other cultures where people do not sleep alone, especially when ill and in need of comfort. Dr. Whiting describes a field trip to Kenya where one of her assistants developed malaria. The villagers sent someone to sleep with and comfort her, since it was understood that someone in physical pain needed physical comfort.

can be expected to affect women in a distinctive way. In both, there is the focus on separation and autonomy which, as we have seen, has different meanings for men and women.

First, it is important to differentiate the issues confronted in adolescence from mid-life transitions and not simply view mid-life changes in adolescent terms. The adolescent crisis of separation from family and commitment to choices differs from the mid-life reassessment of choices which have already been made and shaped over life. The mid-life perspective of finiteness contrasts with the adolescent perspective of an infinite time ahead. The adolescent characteristically deals with ambivalence by externalizing problems and structuring alternatives as mutually exclusive, or by seeking romantic or utopian solutions which promise an escape from conflict. The adult needs to bring a different understanding to bear on problems and the possibilities for their resolution, an understanding which allows for ambiguity, conflict, and ambivalence (Gilligan and Notman, 1978).

For women, the interpretation of mid-life issues in adolescent terms is prevalent since the "two career" lifestyle has been becoming more accepted—with children first and "freedom" second. It is, however, particularly problematic, since female adolescence and development have hitherto been understood in male terms, in which the establishment of identity is thought of as separate from relationships. However, for women, their embeddedness in relationships is well-established. It is, therefore, far from clear what is meant by "autonomy." The comparison and confusion of the concepts of autonomy, "separateness," aloneness, isolation, independence and maturity are far from ended.

Gilligan's (1977) research suggests that women construe moral problems differently from men and that this different moral understanding is tied to a different conception of the relationship between self and others. Women's moral judgments are focused on issues of responsibility, that is, issues involving connections to others rather than abstract rights whose reference is always to the separate self. Because women tend to see people in terms of relationships, issues of competitive achievement look different to them and may be judged differently by them. When achievement enhances the self at the expense of others, women may judge such achievement as "selfish" and regard it as "immoral." This has a bearing on problems arising in relation to careers and their requirements, especially careers entered in mid-life.

CAREER PROBLEMS

The more traditional pattern, at least for middle-class women, has been for women to marry and have children first; then, when the children reach school age or older, the woman returns to work or develops a career interest or perhaps returns to school. As we have seen, many of these patterns are changing. Career-oriented women have been establishing themselves in work first, then making decisions about children. Economic necessity has also led many women to work when their children are small, sometimes without significant interruptions. Divorce and single-parent families with consequent financial pressures contribute to the increase in these changing patterns of women's work.

When a woman has been the central family caretaker and then makes a more serious work or career commitment, family strains result and require adaptation. Women who have previously been the major providers of nurturance in their families then have less time, attention, and may be less sensitive and available. Husbands, even if they are supportive of their wives' working, may react with anger, depression, or other expressions of stress. Children also respond to these changes and their reactions or possible problems may affect the self-esteem of the women, which is often vulnerable in any case. Conflicts about achievement, morality, and selfishness result for the woman. To function effectively in her work may require a degree of aggressiveness which is in conflict with the woman's concept of herself as feminine, or as a loving, caring person (Nadelson, Notman, and Bennett, 1978).

"Assertiveness training" and "leadership training" programs have been springing up to help women overcome their internal barriers and conflicts arising from free expression of a kind of assertiveness which may be necessary for effective work. These are sometimes helpful, but are also symptomatic of existing difficulties.

Conflicts about aggression may be resolved by repression, displacement, avoidance, regression or a variety of other defenses. Ironically, the inhibition of aggression or other defenses adopted unconsciously in order not to hurt others by direct expression of aggression may result in a depression which does hurt everyone indirectly. It is often difficult to separate neurotic conflicts from reality conflicts in the lives of women because there are realistic barriers and angry counterresponses to aggressiveness as well as to failure to perform. In attempts to sort out the realistic from the neurotic, one also encounters the tendency for women to equate achievement of "autonomy" with "separateness" rather than freedom of choice. Maintenance or reliance upon relationships is equated with "dependency." This focus on "separation" as equivalent to maturity creates a view of adult life as a series of passages to be traveled alone and ignores the mutuality of mature adult interdependence. Autonomy requires the sense of one's own boundaries rather than aloneness.

It is possible to see in the particular nature of women's experience a clear direction for understanding adult development. Autonomy and care can be seen not as antithetical, but rather as mutually enhancing. This would involve an acceptance of conflict as internal and ambivalence as inevitable to some degree, and also acknowledgment of reality, rather than relying on the adolescent externalization of conflict and ambivalence and seeing problems as resolvable by making external choices.

It is the nature of the conflict between caring and autonomy which imparts a distinctive character to women's life cycle and determines the particular constraints which women face at mid-life. While women repeatedly have trouble with issues of individuation and separation, these troubles emerge not only from conflicts over aggression but also from women's traditional and universal assumption and valuing of caring and nurturant roles. At mid-life, these roles are inevitably undergoing change, and these changes occur in the context of possibilities which become limited. While some of these limitations are clearly culturally determined and thus subject to change, others are biologically fixed, or rooted in what may be deeply established psychological differences in male and female patterns. Women thus enter mid-life with a different history and relationship between autonomy and relatedness. While the integration of autonomy and caring is a major task of adult development for both sexes, there are real constraints in the timing of this integration for women because of their biological timetable. If such an integration has not developed before mid-life, the opportunities for realizing it are severely diminished (Gilligan and Notman, 1978).

Because choices of love and work in adult life are problematic in a particular way for women, the mid-life reassessment of these choices can be expected to take a somewhat different form than for men. For men, there is a direct connection between self-assertion in the form of achievement (work) and connections to others (love). Since independent self-assertion is socially supported in men, particularly by women, it enhances sexual attraction and leads to opportunities for relationships. At mid-life, the man who has reached a high level of personal achievement has thereby increased his possibilities for relationships with women. For women, however, assertion is a conflicted experience which appears to threaten femininity. Rather than enhancing attractiveness, independence and success on the part of women have often been considered to endanger their relationships.

The reality is that time is limited and that although choices do exist or even increase, there is also a limited range and variety of careers, of new physical pursuits, of new relationships. Yet the possibilities for expansion also exist. The potential for greater autonomy, for changes in relationships and for the development of occupational skills, contracts and expanded self-image may receive a major impetus after childbearing is over. However, further research is needed about women's adult development in a variety of life circumstances, with fewer assumptions about the phases which they are experiencing, and at the same time adequate attention to the implications of their reproductive life stage.

REFERENCES

BARNETT, R. and BARUCH, G.: Women in the middle years: A critique of research and theory. *Psychology of Women Quarterly*, 1978, 3 (2):187-197.

BART, P. & GROSSMAN, M.: Menopause. In M. Notman and C. Nadelson (Eds.), *The Woman Patient*. New York: Plenum Press, 1978.

BENEDEK, T.: Climaterium: A developmental phase. *Psychoanalytic Quarterly*, 1950, 19 (1):1-27.

BUTLER, R.: The facade of chronological age. *American Journal of Psychiatry*, 1963, 119 (8):721-728.

DEUTSCH, H.: *Motherhood: The Psychology of Women*, (Vol. 2): New York: Grune and Stratton, Inc., 1949.

ERIKSON, E. H.: *Childhood and Society* (2nd. Ed.). New York: W. W. Norton, 1963.

FOOTE, A.: Kids who won't leave home. *The Atlantic*, March, 1978, 118.

FRIEDMAN, E. Pregnancy. In M. Notman and C. Nadelson (Eds.), *The Woman Patient*. New York: Plenum Press, 1978.

FREUD, S.: Femininity. In J. Strachey (Ed. and trans.), *New Introductory Lectures in Psychoanalysis*. New York: Norton, 1965. (Originally published, 1933.)

GIELE, J. *Adulthood as Transcendence of Age and Sex*. Paper prepared for the Conference on Love and Work in Adulthood, sponsored by the American Academy of Arts and Sciences, Stanford, CA:, May, 1977.

GILLIGAN, C.: In a different voice: Women's concept of the self and morality. *Harvard Educational Review*, 1977, 47 (4):481-517.

GILLIGAN, C. & NOTMAN, M.: *The Recurrent Theme in Women's Lives: The Integration of Autonomy and Care*. Paper presented at the Eastern Sociological Meetings, Philadelphia, PA., March, 1978.

GOULD, R.: The phases of adult life: A study in developmental psychology. *American Journal of Psychiatry*, 1972, 129 (5):521-531.

KOHLBERG, L.: Sex differences in morality. In E. E. Maccoby (Ed.), *Sex Role Development*. New York: Research Council, 1964.

LEVINSON, D. J., with DARROW, C. N., KLEIN, E. B., LEVINSON, M. H., & McKEE, B.: *The Seasons of a Man's Life*. New York: Knopf, 1978.

LOEVINGER, J.: *Ego Development*. San Francisco: Jossey-Bass Publishers, 1976.

MASTERS, W. H. & JOHNSON, V. E.: *Human Sexual Response*. Boston: Little, Brown & Co., 1966.

McKINLEY, S. & McKINLEY, J.: Selected studies on the menopause. *Journal of Biosocial Science*, 1973, 5:533-555.

McKINLEY, S. & JEFFERYS, M.: The menopausal syndrome. *British Journal of Preventive and Social Medicine*, 1974, 28 (2):108-115.

McKINLEY, S., JEFFERYS, M., & THOMPSON, B.: An investigation of the age at menopause. *Journal of Biosocial Science*, 1972, 4:161-173.

MILLER, J. B. *Towards a New Psychology of Women*. Boston: Beacon Press, 1976.

NADELSON, C., NOTMAN, M., & BENNETT, M.: Success or failure: Psychotherapeutic considerations for women in conflict. *American Journal of Psychiatry*, 1978, 135 (9): 1092-1096.

NEUGARTEN, B.: The awareness of middle age. In B. Neugarten (Ed.), *Middle Age and Aging*. Chicago: University of Chicago Press, 1968.

NEUGARTEN, B.: Adult personality: Towards a psychology of the life cycle. In W. Sze (Ed.), *Human Life Cycle*. New York: Aronson, 1975.

NEUGARTEN, B.: *Time, Age and the Life Cycle*. Paper presented as a special lecture at the American Psychiatric Association Annual Meeting, Atlanta, Ga., May, 1978.

NEUGARTEN, B. & DATAN, N.: The middle years. In S. Arieti (Ed.), *American Handbook of Psychiatry*, (2nd ed.), Vol. 1. New York: Basic Books, 1974.

NEUGARTEN, B. & KRAINES, R. J.: Menopausal symptoms in women of various ages. *Psychosomatic Medicine*, 1965, 27:266-273.

NEUGARTEN, B., WOOD, V., KRAINES, R., & LOOMIS, B.: Women's attitudes towards menopause. In B. Neugarten (Ed.), *Middle Age and Aging*. Chicago: University of Chicago Press, 1968.

NOTMAN, M.: Is there a male menopause? In L. Rose (Ed.), *The Menopause Book*. New York: Hawthorn Books, 1977.

NOTMAN, M.: *Adult Life Cycles: Changing Hormones and Changing Roles*. Paper presented at the Conference of the Bio-Psychological Factors Influencing Sex Role Related Behaviors, Smith College, Northampton, Ma., Oct. 9-10, 1976.

ORTNER, S.: Is female to male as nature is to culture? In M. Rosaldo and L. Lamphere (Eds.), *Women, Culture and Society*. California: Stanford University Press, 1974.

OSOFSKY, H. J. & SEIDENBERG, P.: Is female menopausal depression inevitable? *Obstetrics and Gynecology*, 1970, 34:611-615.

PARLEE, M.: Social factors in psychology of menstruation: Birth and menopause. *Primary Care*, 1976, 3:477-490.

PERLMUTTER, J.: Temporary symptoms and permanent changes in the menopause. In L. Rose (Ed.), *The Menopause Book*. New York: Hawthorn Books, 1977.

PERLMUTTER, J.: The menopause: A gynecologist's view. In M. Notman and C. Nadelson (Eds.), *The Woman as a Patient*. New York: Plenum Press, 1978.

PRICE, J.: *You're Not Too Old to Have a Baby*. New York: Farrar, Straus, & Giroux, 1977.

REYNOLDS, S.: Physiological and psychogenic factors in the menopausal flush syndrome. In W. Kroger (Ed.), *Psychosomatic Obstetrics, Gynecology and Endocrinology*. Springfield: Charles C Thomas, 1962.

ROSSI, A.: Transition to parenthood. *Journal of Marriage and the Family*, 1968, 38 (1).

SONTAG, S.: The double standard of aging. *Saturday Review*, September 23, 1972, p. 29.

WEISSMAN, M. & KLERMAN, G.: Sex differences and the epidemiology of depression. *Archives of General Psychiatry*, 1977, 34:98-111.

WINOKUR, G.: Depression in the menopause. *American Journal of Psychiatry*, 1973, 130 (1):92-93.

ZILBACH, J.: Family development. In J. Marmor (Ed.), *Modern Psychoanalysis*. New York: Basic Books, 1968.

ZILBACH, J.: *Some Family Developmental Considerations of Mid-life*. Paper presented at the American Psychiatric Association Annual Meeting, New look at mid-life years. Anaheim, Ca., May, 1975.

Chapter 7

Sexual Problems:
Changes and Choices
in Mid-Life

Robert E. Gould

The field of gerontology has only recently become respectable—in the sense that mental health professionals are finally acknowledging developmental patterns associated with the aging process. Unfortunately, the aged are often looked upon as "crocks" for whom little can be done and in whom little interest is shown. Mid-life is, of course, not late life, but mid-life does border on late life and, until recently, our knowledge about this phase within the life cycle has been very limited. The subject of aging—the entire process of aging—was to be avoided, even while it was happening to us.

There was a phrase, quite popular once: Life begins at 40. But that was a whistle in the dark, because the pervasive attitude was that life after 40 was the beginning of the end. More recently, in the 1960s, there was another popular slogan: "Don't trust anyone over 30." This phrase had far greater significance in its time, and more influence on our youth-obsessed culture. It has been a long time since we trusted anyone over 30 or 40—including ourselves. However, as the chapters of this book suggest, we are beginning to recognize mid-life or middle adulthood as an important developmental period within the life cycle.

But why has mid-life suddenly become so fascinating? Our culture's main emphasis, after all, is still on youth. A man in his middle 40s, for instance, is often considered to be at the height of his powers, professionally and financially close to his peak. His consorting with women in their 20s and 30s scarcely raises an eyebrow. A woman in her middle 40s, on the other hand, is often thought to be "over the hill." The idea of her being attracted to, or attractive to, men in their 20s and 30s is still almost scandalous. The culture simply does not approve. Sybil Burton, for example, was accorded sympathy when Richard Burton left her for Elizabeth Taylor. But when she made a new liaison with a much younger man, the press and the public turned on her and attacked her in an emotional way, reflecting the rigid traditional mores of "ageism" in the sexual relationship.

Furthermore, it is apparent that in this culture we still worship the young and the beautiful—Hollywood stars, fashion models draped over new cars, and the Pepsi generation. Although we permit an occasional older hero, a sincere, long-standing star such as Henry Fonda or Joe DiMaggio, to sell us a car or a coffee machine, our heroes, our symbols, are still mostly our juniors. As discussed in more detail by Dr. Gutmann in Chapter 3 of this volume, we do not as a society revere our elders for their wisdom and experience. We have never had a rich cultural tradition of respecting or acknowledging this phase within the life cycle as a potential period for development. Instead, we have fostered a tradition which regards older people as useless and used up. Until very recently, for instance, retirement age in almost all work areas steadily declined from 65 to 60 and even to 55. Now, as our population has begun to age, we are finally seeing a backlash against this trend, a revolution by able-bodied men and women dedicated to returning the retirement age not only back to 65, but to 70 and beyond. This is a sudden and dramatic change. What are some of the reasons for it?

At the turn of the century and for several decades thereafter, the average life span for both men and women was considerably shorter than it is today. Not only did many women die in childbirth, but both men and women often succumbed to various diseases which could not be controlled or treated. Those who did survive into mid-life and beyond were "older" than their years—compared to today's standards. Of equal significance was the fact that the typical marriage at that time was never made to last 50 years. The typical marriage at that time was never made to last 50 years. The average marriage lasted about 15 to 20 years before one of the spouses died. Today we are faced with vast numbers of middle-aged marriages, healthy 40- to 50-year-old men and women, who have been married 15 to 20 years, whose children are grown and out of the home and in many cases out of the lives of their parents. With improved living conditions, more affluence and increased longevity, the major emphasis in mid-life marriage has shifted from worry about survival and economic security to concern for the quality of married life—whether the basic needs for love, understanding, and companionship are being met, and if not, what can be done about it.

Similarly, in more recent years we have come to recognize the price paid for trends such as early retirement and enforced leisure. The dream of golden sunset years in a home or "retirement community," aggressively sold by Madison Avenue as a perfect and happy ending for our "senior citizens" is, of course, an American myth. Clinically, we have seen individuals forced into retirement and lacking inner resources for an idle life; once their work lives ceased, their capacity for life in general also decreased. In Hollywood movies, boy met girl, they fought for eight reels, and finally realized they loved each other, despite having little in common. In Hollywood, as in fairytales—not only for children, but for grown-ups—living "happily ever after" was simply what people did. We were never supposed to wonder what that "ever after" life was like on a daily basis. Today, we have begun to examine that life. We can no longer ignore the fact that more of us are in better health and living longer—even if not happily. In light of the above observations and the consequence of recent social changes and concomitant changes in the life cycle, such as increased longevity, we are at last becoming more aware of the developmental changes of the middle years.

One of these is an increasing awareness of the discrepancy between traditional sex roles and the culture's current emphasis on companionship and equality within the sexual relationship. The sex-role changes that occur in mid-life, like other transitions in the life cycle, are a product of multiple determinants and, in part at least, contingent upon the manner in which the psychosexual challenges of previous phases of development were mastered. As noted by Dr. Lidz in Chapter 2, one's development, at whatever phase of the life cycle, is the summation and integration of all previous identifications and experiences. For example, the capacity for intimacy and interdependence with one's partner depends to a large extent on the intrafamilial, socioeconomic and cultural experiences which provide the consistency that characterizes an individual, despite changes that occur over time and also despite the many different roles assumed at any one period of life. If sex is determined by biological imperatives, the role ascribed to one's sex is determined by cultural norms within the broad context bounded by biology. Each individual in the culture responds sexually not only in terms of sexual drive, but in terms of the interpersonal implications which such actions have been given (Mead, 1949).

This chapter focuses on the sexual challenges confronting middle-aged adults and examines the extent to which previous psychosexual experiences influence future sex-role conflicts.

To illustrate this point, it may be helpful to examine the past lives of current mid-lifers so that we can focus clearly on their present predicament. How did our two middle-aged mates, who are 50 today, grow up? Our sexist society needs no documentation, but an understanding of our sexist roots is crucial to any analysis of the psychosexual challenges and sex-role conflicts that confront our current mid-life generation. When today's 50-year-olds were children, boys and girls grew up along two distinct and separate tracks. There were different expectations for the male and female, and different views of appropriate "masculine" and "feminine" behavior. Even before birth, when blue was chosen for the boys' nursery, and pink for the girls', the die was being cast: The two sexes were to be treated, raised and regarded as distinctly different species. After birth, the message became louder, clearer, and more constant. Adults tended to hold baby girls more gently, to encourage small boys not to cry, to approve of doll-play for girls, and to expect more aggressivity in boys. Boys learned to be ambitious and more career-oriented, while girls of the last two generations were socialized for marriage, home, and motherhood. The dream of every girl was marked by a white picket fence—around a house full of children and a tired husband. If we view films as a cultural barometer, it is interesting to note that the movies of the past taught the country, as television does today, that even the redoubtable "career girl" played by Rosalind Russell or Katharine Hepburn, quit her job when she met the right man who could tame her or bring out her "femininity." The all-American heroine was a woman who married and accepted the wifely role (and the second-class status) that Freud, if not God, had ordained for her. According to Freud (1963), women must come to accept their secondary status and compensate for their deficits (i.e. lack of a penis) by having a baby and a husband (Gould, 1975). Although Freud assumed that the major difference in role function between men and women was based on biology and anatomy and, therefore, inevitable and universal, the current evidence suggests that the role difference between the sexes is primarily induced by cultural attitudes, rather than by any biological givens (Gould, 1975). Two of the best-known and respected names in the psychoanalytic business today—Erik H. Erikson and Bruno Bettelheim—however, still hold that a woman's primary role as mother and homemaker must be fulfilled before she turns to other interests.

When today's middle-aged couple were children, tradition demanded that boys play with boys; if they showed interest in girls or girls' games they were called sissies or worse—queers. It was apparent that boys had little respect for girls, and did not make friends with them. During the critical juvenile and preadolescent periods, friendships, collaborative efforts and the process of learning to share intimacies all developed on a same-sex basis—never between boys and girls (Sullivan, 1953).

At the onset of adolescence, with surging hormones providing the biological urge, the culture again defined and directed boy-girl interaction. The adolescent boy was expected to make his first fumbling sexual overtures in the back seat of a car, the back row of the movie balcony, or under the grandstand of a high school football field. The nice girl was not to say yes, but neither could she say "no" too firmly. Everyone was trained to play a role; the dance of "love" was choreographed as meticulously as a minuet—with little room for spontaneity or individual expression. The final step in this dance was, of course, marriage, the only sociably approved ending for the sexual liaison. Marriage signified that both boy and girl had grown up, and now were ready to perform their adult roles—the woman anchored and given her well-structured, life long position of homemaker; the man venturing forth to conquer the world, or at least to bring home the bacon.

The main problem with this scenario, besides the obvious one that men and women were rigidly programmed for these social roles, was the relatively low value placed on companionship and mutuality in sexual relations. The outcome of this scenario can be seen, then, as an extension of a more generalized developmental pattern. The separate paths that boys and girls travelled on the way to adulthood all but ruled out the possibility of closeness and companionship. One of the sad effects of sexism is that real intimacy between the sexes, founded on respect and friendship, becomes extremely difficult to achieve. It is understandable that husbands and wives may not think of sexual relations as a way of relating intimately when they have so few reasons for doing so. The traditional sex-role segregation, of which the pattern of sexual relations seems a part, has, as one consequence, problems in communication between husbands and wives on matters not clearly defined in terms of traditional expectations (Balswick and Peek, 1975). It is extremely difficult for such couples to cope with problems which require mutual accommodation and empathy. A generation ago, we did not have marriages between equals or couples who respected each other as peers. This may be one reason why many husbands quickly opted for their nights out with the boys—poker games, fishing trips, and hanging out at a favorite bar. This pattern of married male behavior is beautifully dissected in James Dickey's book *Deliverance,* in which the "he-men" escaped from their marriages to shoot the rapids and court dangerous adventure together. It was an accepted truth that men could "be themselves" only with other men—their drinking, hunting, cursing, girl-chasing buddies. It was frequently assumed that only homosexual men could be "friends" with women.

In the movies of the 1960s and 70s, this tradition reached its ultimate extreme, in the frequent pairing of two virile male stars whose real love interest seemed to be each other. Paul Newman and Robert Redford, Jack Nicholson and Peter Fonda, Dustin Hoffman and Jon Voight, Elliot Gould and Donald Sutherland are examples. Their he-man adventures were, of course, logical civilian extensions of the old war movies, in which buddies were true to each other, would die for each other, and sealed their loyalty through honor, heroism, and intimacies far beyond those a man could share with any woman. Romantic love for a woman—the sexual connection— was made to seem as exciting momentary diversion from the real stuff of a man's life—his bonding with other men.

By the early 1970s, women had all but disappeared from the scene. Although an occasional girl flitted past as a transient sex object (to prove that the buddy-heroes were red-blooded heterosexuals), there were no fully developed female roles. On television, there were mothers in shows called Father Knows Best, and wives who kept various home-fires burning. But even on television, the action-adventure shows, westerns, and spy mysteries were primarily set in a man's world, where women appeared only as passing sex objects, with no other claim for the hero's or the audience's attention.

For the first time in perhaps a decade, we have begun to see a break in this tradition. Movies and television shows are beginning to revolve around female stars as fully developed characters. Recent films, such as *Julia, A Turning Point,* and *An Unmarried Woman,* represent intense studies of women and the complex emotional interaction between the sexes. Moreover, these films highlight early landmarks in our changing cultural landscape, and portray American life in an actual sexual revolution. The revolution is, of course, far from over. Indeed, we are in the thick of the battle, and the casualty list continues to mount among all age groups, though most dramatically among the mid-life generation—who developed under rigidly defined sexual norms and polarized sex roles. While the women struggled vainly to conform to the prevailing image of themselves as totally passive, not-quite-human beings, men fought to fuse the many conflicting cultural signals for ideal masculine behavior. That is, they sought to be strong, independent, aggressive, tough, loyal to each other, but also highly competitive. To be a man, one could never reveal deep emotions, especially fears, anxieties or anything that could be construed as being "weak" or "feminine." Men who felt less competitive, or needed to express their deeper feelings, could only do so with a woman they perceived as "understanding and non-threatening."

It seems unlikely that today's male mid-lifer ever really loved any woman, including his spouse, in the sense that love means a mature, mutually gratifying sexual relationship between two people who respect each other as equals. What passed for love in the early years of our mid-lifers' marriages was a combination of lust and the romantic idealizing that we were taught to invest in the person we chose to marry. It is a small wonder that when romance and lust subside, as they inevitably do, the couple drifts apart because neither party is accustomed to relating intimately with the other. For many middle-aged couples, particularly in the middle-class, the mid-life period is a point of maximum involvement in careers, family, child rearing, and other diversions which prevent both partners from recognizing how little remains of the marriage. The raising of children, all the homemaking and maintenance activities of the wife, and the career pursuits of the husband create a climate of busyness that often clouds the reality of how little actually exists between the partners. For many couples, "marriage" becomes a "form" with little substance. It is not uncommon at this time for either spouse to engage in excessive drinking, extramarital affairs and other distractions as consolation for the emptiness of the marriage. Offer and Simon (1975) report that over one-half of all men and about one-fourth of all women report at least one extramarital affair during this period. For both sexes, patterning of extramarital sexual activity continues to be expressive of earlier patterns of psychosexual development. The man retains his old capacity for detachment which in adolescence was directly related to the pursuit of sexual fantasies and the social validation of masculinity. For women, on the other hand, the pursuit of an affair resembles a quest for circumstances that justify and confirm a romantic self-image, rather than a quest for lost orgasms.

But once the children are out of the home and the husband has gone about as far as he will go in his job, the couple is confronted with a new crisis—one of the few times in their marriage in which there is time for reflection and evaluation of their lives. This is the point at which many couples find they have little in common, little to share, and little mutual respect. Communication problems that have been hidden become vividly apparent. It is my opinion that many of our traditional sex-role expectations limit the development of intrapersonal and interpersonal potentials and are out of step with contemporary society which emphasizes flexibility, companionship and equality within the relationship.

Today's typical 50-year-old male has other problems as well. He has lived most of his life in a competitive world where his status and prestige have been based on external values (i.e., what people think of him, his job title, salary, friends, and status in general) rather than internal values (i.e., a feeling of self-esteem and self-worth based on the kind of person he knows he is). In late middle age, aproximately 55, he begins to feel depressed, scared, and unsure of himself as he realizes that he is no longer young, vigorous or upwardly mobile. These feelings have always been more acute in women, but increasingly, men too have begun to succumb to them. It is interesting to note that commercials on television are selling cosmetics and other articles (e.g., dyes for men's hair), once the sole province of women, to a rapidly increasing male clientele. The cultural emphasis on youth is still strong, and the typical macho male still places great value on his potency and virility, which he regards as virtually synonymous with manhood.

Yet we know, and the evidence is incontrovertible, that man's greatest sexual capacity, if measured by the quantity of ejaculations, peaks at age 17 or 18. By age 45 or 50, there is a noticeable decrease in sexual capacity which may threaten a man's confidence in his verility. If the quality of the marital relationship is poor, he may find himself sexually dysfunctional with his spouse. To prove himself, he may, on occasion, seek younger women to reaffirm his waning sexual power. This pattern may, however, cause additional performance deficits and/or anxiety, since he is physically less capable of sustained sexual activity. An additional source of stress for the middle-aged adult, which may affect the sexual responsiveness of both partners, is the fear of losing one's partner to a younger and more attractive person.

A clinical example might help to illustrate some of the issues that confront middle-aged couples and also the extent to which given difficulties are specifically age-related or derivatives of earlier psychosexual developmental challenges.

A middle-aged couple came for treatment because of marital discord. James H., age 50, and his wife, Jane, age 45, have three grown children, two of whom have left the home. James is a successful stockbroker and senior partner in his firm. Jane, on the other hand, committed herself to the wife/mother role, keeping her days filled with little things, but empty of anything real or fulfilling. The couple married soon after college; within a few years, James acquired a mistress whom he set up in a Manhattan apartment, while maintaining his family in a fashionable suburban home.

In the course of therapy, it became evident that sexism and respect for one's mate are simply incompatible. Through his affairs and management of them, James was continuously trying to reassure himself that he was attractive, powerful, and successful. So long as the women in his life did not demand commitment, he could feel comfortable and secure that he was achieving his idea of "manhood," but on a deeper level he could never really believe it. Each liaison broke up for a different reason. With one partner, he became bored because the relationship was basically only a sexual one. Another failed when the woman felt that she needed more of his time and wanted marriage. None of James' relationships could be really satisfying in a long-lasting way, because he never could relate to any woman as an equal; eventually she would "fail" him when the romantic period ended. On the other hand, Jane thought that by marrying a rich, energetic, and powerful husband, her life as a wife, mother, and mistress of a lovely home would be all a woman could ask for. However, Jane eventually discovered the emptiness of her relationship. Sometimes bored, sometimes angry or depressed, she took Valium, television, and liquor in about equal doses. Marrying James turned out not to be enough after all, because the marriage, although amicable, was superficial; James simply could not relate to her on an intimate level.

As of now, James is maintaining his uneasy, dual life, guilty and dissatisfied, commuting between his wife, his job and his mistresses. He is "successful," but he cannot understand why nothing makes him happy. Although he and his wife have reached an "understanding," they have apparently agreed to live out their lives in quiet desperation. In this particular example, there are suggestions that the relationship will continue to deteriorate. James is more anxious and sometimes frantic about maintaining his affairs, while Jane, on the other hand, is becoming more snappish with her husband as the demands of her maternal role diminish, leaving her more time to concentrate on James. Her sexual needs are unsatisfied, but her whole past history has made adultery difficult for her. She is beginning to drink and take tranquilizers more frequently.

This case example illustrates the pressures of mid-life and its unbalancing effect on a relatively stable, if not happy, life-style. The picture is not atypical of many middle- and upper-middle-class marriages. For women who married very young and started raising children, or who may have spent a few aimless years in the business world before marriage, home becomes the entire world. Such women have perceived the family's needs as their central focus of life. Where can such a woman turn, what are her options, at age 45, with no career and presumably limited capital assets with which to start a new life? Middle-aged women without independent sources of income often feel trapped into staying with men who may no longer be satisfactory mates. If men their own age look towards younger women, and society still frowns on older women-younger men relationships, the hopelessness of this situation often registers in women's rage, anger, or depression.

Frequently, in this predicament, women are very difficult to treat.

With the children's departure from home and the sense of declining opportunities with advancing age, women experience a significant void and find themselves left only with a marriage that has run dry. Should they try to start a new life in a professional career, they often find they lack the necessary skills and are too old for training in what might be "good jobs." If they pursue separation and divorce, they are often confronted with the fact that unattached men in mid-life are looking for younger women. Even an attractive, intelligent woman in mid-life finds it extremely difficult to find an acceptable new partner of her own age. During mid-life, these women face a new and increasing powerlessness as their former sexual roles become more and more difficult to play. If the middle-aged woman, whose mothering role is also over, has no occupation or other interests, she must look more to her husband for comfort, even as he is looking elsewhere to fulfill his needs.

> Carol, age 45, and John, age 48, came for therapy at the insistence of the wife, who felt helpless in a disintegrating marriage. They had both been married once before, when they were quite young—she to an alcoholic whom she tended for several years before he died in an automobile accident. Carol and John have been married for 15 years. Shortly after marriage, Carol worked briefly as an owner of an antique shop. John showed little interest in her business and she soon gave it up and spent her days aimlessly. She saw friends, played bridge and shopped a good deal. The house was always well-kept and food and drink were plentiful. John, a successful insurance agent, is a heavy drinker, belongs to a country club where he plays golf, drinks and socializes a great deal, usually alone and without his wife's approval. He has had numerous extramarital affairs, two or three of which were more substantial than one-night stands. John often missed dinner; at times he would call to say that he would be home in an hour, and then he would not show up for two or three hours. Although this happened repeatedly, Carol was always there ready to serve him and forgive him. She rarely nagged or complained but played the role of a martyr and certainly fit everyone's definition of a masochist.

> As they unfolded their story, Carol saw herself as having no problems. All she wanted was for John to be more loving and

caring, to stop having affairs and to spend more time with her. John readily admitted that he was totally to blame, everything was his fault; he agreed that Carol was a perfect wife. He felt guilty but did not appear to be motivated to change his ways. In therapy, it was emphasized that the problem was not just the husband's, but also the wife's for putting up with his behavior all these years and for not developing any outlets herself so that she would not be totally dependent upon him emotionally. Her family had left her some money, so that, unlike many wives, she was not completely dependent upon him financially.

John and Carol were seen in group therapy. Their group was composed of men and women who were all dissatisfied with their sex roles and/or their heterosexual relationships. The consensual validation from all members of the group confirmed that Carol was, in part, responsible for their problems because she put up with John's behavior—in fact, she even encouraged it by her passive acceptance. But despite the group's prodding, Carol was unable to become more assertive with John, or to do more to develop her own potential for growth and change. She had played one role for so long, beginning with her first husband and then with John, that she did not have the resources to draw upon to explore other options that might have been available to her. Her commitment to a particular sex-role model was so thorough that she firmly believed that she could not achieve anything on her own. As a couple exhibiting stereotypical male and female traits, John and Carol were a little extreme. For example, John always drove the car when they went out together and if Carol saw a parking space, he would pass it by until he found one himself. He was a macho male with a vengeance. Their sex life had stopped three years prior to their entering therapy, when Carol learned of John's semi-serious affair with another woman. Although she expressed the desire not to resume sex again until he stopped having affairs, her past behavior suggested that, if John had sought sex with her, she would have complied. John, however, was satisfied with the current agreement and perceived her statement as an excuse for him to withdraw from her sexually, particularly since he had lost all romantic feelings for her. His primary reason for remaining with Carol was that she was "nice to come home to," his laundry was ready, his food was always prepared, and she offered a sympathic ear if he needed one.

Therapy failed for John and Carol as a couple. They left the group and, six months later, John left Carol and called to ask if I would see his girl friend, a 27-year-old woman whom he had been seeing when he first came into therapy with his wife. John wanted me to tell the girl friend how bad he was, and to see if she would accept him "as is." I was able to persuade him that this approach was untenable, and that unless he now saw or felt the need for a real change in his life-style, it was doubtful that he would ever build a really gratifying relationship with any woman. He and his girl friend entered therapy as a couple because she was making demands on him that his wife never had made. This may be the impetus John needs to make the changes which are essential to the establishment of anything approaching an equal, satisfying relationship with a woman.

Carol, and other long-suffering wives like her, typify a large group of middle-aged women who are victims of their own deep-seated feelings of rage and helplessness. The new, much publicized climate of freedom to express powerful negative emotions—to "let it all hang out"—does not really help such women, because their anger, often unconscious, cannot be safely vented. The man who would be the likeliest target is most often a husband upon whom the woman is still totally dependent for financial and emotional support. The only other target for the anger is herself—for being powerless to leave, or even to demand drastic changes within the relationship. The prevailing culture, despite a few dramatic signs of change—runaway wives and assertive young brides with "marriage contracts"—continues to inhibit women, in general, from openly displaying aggressivity, or ventilating hostile feelings, even when justified. Thus, the rage is still most often directed inward and converted to depression and/or anxiety. This entrenched emotional pattern helps maintain a multi-million-dollar drug industry. Doctors provide these women with anti-depressants and psychotropic drugs for chemical relief of the anxiety and depression. Somehow this prescription is viewed as preferable to any serious attempt to change the lives of these women—a task that may well seem insurmountable.

The women's movement has had a paradoxical effect, causing some women to become more aware of opportunities wasted, lives lived in frustration and fear of the unknown world outside the home. On the other hand, some women have been helped by the emotional and educative support offered by the women's movement. These women not only welcome the "empty nest" but perceive the mid-life period as providing additional opportunities to pursue personal, educational, and occupational interests. In such women, a new assertiveness can be seen—a restlessness to take on the challenges that they were physically and/or emotionally unable to face before. For such women, mid-life and its challenges offer a renewed opportunity for making a new life with or without a husband.

Sullivan (1953) astutely observed that in periods of transition there is great opportunity for change—for good or for ill.* There are new tasks and opportunities and often a new cast of characters to demand a new way of relating. For those talented or resourceful enough to draw on internal and external reserves, mid-life offers a chance for further development and growth. To be sure, Sullivan was not so naive as to be unaware that one carries the psychological baggage from a previous phase into the next one. If one has been severely hurt or traumatized in an earlier stage of development, it will be more difficult to make use of new options in later life. Although Sullivan never elaborated on the chances for revival and growth during the mid-life period, his whole schema of personality development, which never allows for closure until death, suggests hope for those now facing the strains and challenges of the mid-life period. Erik Erikson, Roger Gould, and Daniel Levinson, in their elaborations of the ways in which later stages of life offer options for change and growth, clearly owe a debt to Sullivan's pioneering work in this area.

In exploring the possibilities for positive change in mid-life, however, it must be noted that the biological changes which naturally occur in this period tend to put nature at odds with cultural conventions. In our culture, the older man who is divorced or widowed frequently seeks a younger woman for a mate, or a mistress if he is still married. If the age difference is great, or if the woman is very young, he may be called a "dirty old man," not always unkindly. However, as noted previously, an older woman who takes up

---

* In discussing the periods of transition, Sullivan's theories of transition focused primarily on childhood to juvenility to preadolescence and following that into the never-never land of maturity.

with a younger man is subject to much sharper social disapproval. Sexuality in an older woman is perceived as embarrassing, if not repugnant. Similarly, mid-life is often accompanied with loss of sex appeal and perhaps the end of serious sexual activity as well. As discussed in more detail by Dr. Notman in Chapter 6 of this volume, the cessation of the menses in women is a biological event which signifies a definite change in the functioning of the body. There is no comparable biological event in men's lives. With no such specific change to mark the man's "menopause" as such, it is generally taken for granted that the man remains sexually active through his 50s and perhaps well into his 60s. Again, if we take movies as a cultural barometer, the older-man, younger-woman romance is commonplace; the reverse is almost never portrayed.

Biologically, the paradox and irony of all of this are that middle-aged women not only experience minimal loss of their capacity to achieve orgasms, but report an actual increase in sexual responsiveness following the cessation of the menses, whereas the man as he ages experiences increasingly lengthened refractory periods. The potential for man's capacity to reach a climax decreases steadily after the late teens, while the woman's ability remains on a virtual plateau throughout her 50s and 60s. In fact, many women who grew up sexually inhibited or repressed currently report finding a new sexual freedom in mid-life. This freedom extends to having love affairs and marriages with men younger than themselves.

The male ego's traditional safety valve—affirming one's masculinity by engaging in sex with younger women—seems to be working less well now. Women are somewhat less attracted to older men's power, money, and status since these achievements can now be sought directly. Rather than faking sexual satisfaction to please and flatter a man, women are becoming more candid and assertive, and less turned on by the man's "superior" social role. Indeed, as she emerges sexually, the younger woman poses as much of a "challenge" or threat as does his contemporary partner (wife).

Some middle-aged men have reacted to the anxiety of the changing sexual roles and sexual attitudes of middle-aged and younger women by retreating to a still younger female—the nymphet, the 12-year-old sex object. This appears to be the only "safe" target left for the frightened middle-aged man. There is a rise in "kiddie porn," incest, and the desire of older men for teen and preteenaged prostitutes. The *Lolita* phenomenon was not unique but a harbinger of things to come. The film *Taxi Driver* featured a teenaged prostitute and *Pretty Baby* lowered the prostitute's age to 12.

The rise in uncommitted sex represents still another aspect of the male backlash against the emergence of strong, assertive women. Men who cannot tolerate the idea of an equal relationship with women continue to retreat into fantasy sex worlds—porn shops, massage parlors, and men's magazines, where women are still docile playthings, and sex is a man's sport. The mainstream, however, seems to be moving in its bumpy, erratic course toward greater equality between the sexes and the possibility of friendship and mutual respect upon which genuine love can be built. The profound change in women's attitudes about themselves has come about through many factors including the Feminist Movement, consciousness-raising groups, self-awareness books, education, etc. This phenomenon has not occurred in a vacuum. Men's attitudes also are continuing to undergo drastic changes. As they begin to view women differently, they must also reexamine their own sex role. As men reexamine the culturally imposed macho posture, and move toward a more androgynous state, some of them are beginning to experience the more emotional, tender, and nurturant qualities in themselves.

This presents a major challenge to psychiatrists, whose therapies will be appropriate and effective only if the practitioners acknowledge and understand the need for the changing sexual roles of men and women and are willing to confront the fact that marriage, in the old, traditional sense, never allowed the partners to develop fully into the individuals they were meant to be. The sexist and anti-aging attitudes of our society have never been adequately acknowledged. Psychiatrists and other mental health professionals must begin to recognize the tremendous influence of such attitudes in compromising the mental health and personality development of both sexes.

The sexual revolution is vastly more complicated than just a matter of giving women equal sexual rights or eliminating the double standard; men and women must reexamine their attitudes toward aging, and their adherence to traditional sex roles which appear to be out of step with changes in contemporary society. As men and women change their thinking about themselves and their commitment to traditional sex roles, they will also change, and perhaps ultimately eliminate, the effects of sexism on the quality of interpersonal relationships.

Psychiatrists and mental health professionals must offer education as well as treatment to help us become a people who can age gracefully without losing our sexual appetites, appeal, or capability. It is equally important that our institutions, which play so large a part in shaping the culture, begin to adapt to the new views of men and women. The church, the educational system, the laws which govern the institution of marriage—all will have to undergo their own revolution, modifying or discarding ideas of "traditional roles" based on gender differences. If middle-age is not to be a crisis period, but one of continued growth for men and women and their relationships, then old values proven false or inadequate to today's men and women must give way to "non-traditional," truly human, roles for men and women as individuals.

REFERENCES

BALSWICK, J. & PEEK, C.: The inexpressive male: A tragedy of American society. In W. Sze (Ed.), *The Human Life Cycle*. New York: Jason Aronson, Inc., 1975.

DEUTSCH, H.: *The Psychology of Women*. New York: Grune & Stratton, 1944.

ERIKSON, E. H.: *Childhood and Society*, (2nd ed.). New York: W. W. Norton, 1963.

FREUD, S.: Female sexuality. In *Standard Edition of the Complete Psychological Works of Sigmund Freud*, Vol. 21. London: Hogarth Press, 1961.

FREUD, S.: The sexual life of human beings. In *Standard Edition of the Complete Psychological Works of Sigmund Freud*, Vol. 16. London: Hogarth Press, 1963.

GOULD, R.: The phases of adult life: A study in developmental psychology. *American Journal of Psychiatry*, 1972, 129 (5):521-531.

GOULD, R.: Sociocultural roles of male and female. In A. Freedman, H. Kaplan, and B. Sadock (Eds.), *Comprehensive Textbook of Psychiatry—II*, (2nd ed.), Vol. 2. Baltimore: Williams & Wilkins Co., 1975.

LEVINSON, D. J., with DARROW, C. N., KLEIN, E. B., LEVINSON, M. H., & McKEE, B.: *The Seasons of Man's Life*. New York: Alfred A. Knopf, 1970.

MEAD, M.: *Sex and Temperament*. New York: New American Library, 1935.

MEAD, M.: *Male and Female*. New York: Morow, 1949.

OFFER, D., & SIMON, W.: Stages of sexual development. In A. Freedman, H. Kaplan, and B. Sadock (Eds.), *Comprehensive Textbook of Psychiatry—II*, (2nd ed), Vol. 2. Baltimore: Williams & Wilkins, Co., 1975.

SULLIVAN, H. S.: *The Interpersonal Theory of Psychiatry*. New York: Norton, 1953.

Chapter 8

Mid-Life and the Family: Strains, Challenges and Options of the Middle Years

Carola H. Mann

Until recently, the professional community has paid little attention to age-related changes in adulthood. Literature and fiction, though acknowledging adulthood and specifically middle age as legitimate topics, tend to emphasize the deprivations associated with middle age. Pejorative jokes about the proverbial middle age spread or the seven year itch predominate over more serious interest in the developmental challenges and accomplishments of the middle years. Even the recent interest in family life and family therapy seems to focus on earlier stages such as the years of childbearing or adolescent turmoil rather than on the strains and challenges of the middle years.

The neglect of family and marital issues in the mid-life years is not altogether surprising in view of the fact that psychology in general has not paid much attention to the middle years of life.

Generally, developmental theories have addressed themselves to the younger individual whose psychological changes parallel physiological developments. Since physiological changes are minimal in adulthood, psychological events in the middle years have been regarded merely as orchestrations of earlier adaptations with little importance of their own. Similarly, as pointed out by Dr. Notman in Chapter 6, the research concerned with the middle years of life has primarily focused on individuals, in particular, men, rather than on the couple and the family. Of equal importance is that both longitudinal (Cox, 1976; Valliant, 1977) and cross-sectional researches (Levinson, Darrow, Klein, Levinson, and McKee, 1974) have seldom investigated the individual past 50 years of age.

If knowledge of the mid-life experience of men and women is limited, research data about the family in the middle years are even less available. Most of the information about this period of life comes from clinical experience where, by necessity, the emphasis is on pathology. In short, while we await support from the research literature, discussion of marriage and the family in the middle years will be based primarily on clinical experience.

THE FAMILY IN THE MIDDLE YEARS

Before examining the issues confronted by the middle-aged couple and its family, it seems appropriate to define middle age. The dictionary defines middle age as "the time of human life between youth and old age, usually reckoned as the years between 40 and 60" (*American Heritage Dictionary*, 1977, p. 830). As discussed in previous chapters of this volume, this definition of middle age is simplistic and only one of several possible definitions (i.e. chronological, physiological, and socio-psychological). It is also important to note that any definition of the mid-life period offers limited information about the issues confronted by the middle-aged couple and the family.

The middle years represent a time when the middle-aged couple's parents are becoming elderly, perhaps requiring increasing care and certainly increasing concern. On the other end of the generation continuum is the increasing emancipation of the young. Parents, though their financial support is often still required, find themselves bypassed as the younger generation makes important decisions regarding life-styles and career choices, often without consulting them. The younger generation almost by definition has more choices and options than parents do at this time, and the middle-aged parent has to deal with envy and resentment, feelings that stir up guilt and anxiety.

As the middle-aged partners find themselves increasingly alone with one another, they may have to develop a level of intimacy and relatedness that differs from earlier experiences of closeness. To some extent they "meet" for the first time, having mainly traveled separate paths during 20 years of career building and family raising when most shared communications tended to be about children and household matters.

The extent to which each partner in the middle years can accept his or her spouse as an individual with individual interests depends on the possibility of developing a common ground of caring and mutual support for one another, and on developing common interests and yet respecting each other's individuality and separateness.

One way of viewing the middle years and their impact on marriage and family life is to see them as a time that requires changes in relatedness and intimacy, changes that reflect an altered sense of self that is part and parcel of the developmental process of the middle years. Levenson defines intimacy as "the ability to achieve an authentic relationship" which involves a "frank experiencing of one another with awareness and without pressure to change into something else or something better" (Levenson, 1974, p. 363). According to him, the ability to achieve an authentic relationship is an inherent aspect of maturity and thus is of relevance in the context of this chapter.

It is my contention that strains, options, and challenges faced by the family in the middle years of life can best be understood by examining the changed sense of self that characterizes the experience of middle age and that affects interpersonal relationships and expectations in terms of spouses, children, parents, and friends.

THE CHANGING SENSE OF SELF IN THE MIDDLE YEARS*

The changing sense of self in the middle years is reflected in the kind of issues the typical middle-aged individual has to deal with. Although these issues are interrelated, they can be divided for clarity's sake into "self-issues" (i.e. issues that affect primarily one's perception of oneself) and "other-issue" (i.e. issues that refer to specific relationships with significant others). Self-issues include concerns about appearance and physical stamina, work or career, illness, death and dying, amount of time left to live and concerns with one's sexuality. Other-issues refer to relatedness to one's aging parents, relatedness to growing children, and relatedness to mate, peers, and friends.

Physical and Physiological Aging

The middle-aged person is aware of changes in appearance and energy level. Greying hair, weight gain, greater difficulty in recuperating from physical exertion are just a few of the physiological indices of aging. Research confirms the increasing concern with physical appearance and vigor in the middle years (Gould, 1972; Havighurst, 1973). Levinson et al. (1974) report concerns with bodily decline among men in their early 40s; the same concerns are described by Neugarten (1969), who refers to sensitivity to bodily effectiveness at mid-life. Physiological signs of aging are experienced as narcissistic injury by both men and women, although the psychological impact of this injury varies from individual to individual. It is furthermore important to note that women experience the physical aspects of aging primarily as a threat to their attractiveness to men; men are concerned with the extent to which aging puts them at a competitive disadvantage in work and sports (Mann, 1977a).

In the work arena, the typical middle-aged man experiences the threat of the younger competitor; he is aware of the wish to "become his own man" (Levinson et al., 1974) and he is perhaps dissatisfied

* Discussion of mid-life issues is based in part on data collected by means of the Mid-Life Issues Test (MLIT) developed by Lionells and Mann as part of the Mid-Life Research Project at the William Alanson White Institute of Psychiatry, Psychoanalysis, and Psychology.

because he believes that he may have made the wrong career choice early in life (Brown, 1972; Terkel, 1974). At times, mid-life work evaluations lead to career changes for the male.

Women approach work and career questions in the middle years from a different perspective. Since they may have been primarily mothers and homemakers for the preceding 20 years, potential entry into the working world creates a kind of panic that can be likened to separation anxiety. For both men and women, the motivation for vocational changes in the middle years seems related to what has been called in German "Torschlusspanik"*—i.e., the fear that it may be too late to accomplish some of the things one had hoped to accomplish in one's lifetime.

Concerns with Illness, Death and Dying

The middle years also bring with them increasing experience with illness and death as it occurs among parents, parent-surrogates such as teachers and mentors, and among contemporaries. The reality of physical decline and increasing physical limitations brings into sharp relief the reality of one's own mortality and finiteness (Farrell, 1975; Levinson et al., 1974; Marmor, 1974; Schecter and Lippman, 1974). Again men and women differ in their response to issues like death and illness. Men react with anger to the realization that illness and death are inescapable realities of life; women on the other hand seem less anxious about the increasing dependence of elderly friends and relatives. They are more clearly identified with the caretaking role and less conflicted about their own dependency, a dependency that may become more appropriate as they become older (Mann, 1977b).

Time Left to Live

Death and mortality become increasingly real to men and women in their middle years. By necessity, therefore, they have to come to grips with their own finiteness and mortality. Middle age appears to be a time where an individual's concerns shift from time since birth

---

*Torschlusspanik is a German term for "Fear that the gates are closing." It originated in the Middle Ages when the weary traveler had to reach the nearest town before the city gates were closing so as not to be at the mercy of bandits and wild animals.

to time left to live (Clausen, 1972; Neugarten, 1969; Soddy and Kidson, 1967; Terkel, 1974). The "life review" of the middle-aged individual, according to Clausen (1972), is undertaken to integrate experiences and to evaluate one's performance so far in order to improve future performance. Jacques (1965) suggests a similar psychological intrapsychic review when he describes the reworking of earlier disappointments and frustrations.

Sexuality

Psychologically, mid-life men and women undergo changes in sexuality that to some extent take opposing directions and that reflect changes in the activity/passivity dimensions of personality. Women in the middle years tend to shift from a more dependent stance to one that emphasizes development of their own abilities in a more active sense (Back, 1971). Men move from an instrumental mode of interaction to an emphasis on the more feminine aspects of self, such as expressed tenderness, gentleness, a need for security, and an awareness of the feelings of others (Lowenthal, Thurnher, and Chiriboga, 1975). This shift in the activity/passivity dimension is replicated in the sexual area as well, where the middle-aged man frequently begins to experience some loss of potency and slowing down of sexual responsiveness; at the same time, the woman becomes considerably more sexually active and responsive than before the mid-life period (Gadpaille, 1975; Sheehy, 1976). Recent research in sexuality at mid-life stresses the notion that men and women in their mid-life years are sexually "out of phase" (Gadpaille, 1975; Kaplan, 1974). Sexual relationships therefore frequently become a focus of concern and disturbance for the middle-aged couple.

Interpersonal Relationships in the Middle Years

The experience of seeing one's parents becoming dependent is a crucial aspect of the mid-life experience (Farrell, 1975; Havighurst, 1973; Levinson et al., 1974). It contributes to a change in one's sense of self since childhood fantasies of being taken care of need to be reevaluated and worked through in the light of the very concrete role reversal that can take place in the adult years.

At the other end of the generation continuum, the middle years are characterized by what has been called the "empty nest" syndrome (Lowenthal et al., 1975). Previously only the theme of loss had been stressed in reference to the departure of children from the home (Marmor, 1974; Jacques, 1965; Schecter and Lippman, 1974). More recently, however, a theme of freedom, particularly for women, is beginning to emerge when the departure of growing children is being discussed (Back, 1971; Lowenthal et al., 1975; Sheehy, 1976).

As relationships with family members undergo extensive changes in the mid-life period, relatedness patterns and needs also undergo changes (Gould, 1972; Havighurst, 1973; Lionells and Mann, 1978; Lowenthal et al., 1975; Schlossberg, 1966). The mid-life individual seems to place renewed importance on those aspects of living that have to do with a sense of self-fulfillment. The thrust towards self-fulfillment is experienced within the context of being aware and respectful of the needs of others, and particularly of that one person one is closest to (Lionells and Mann, 1978). This, however, is also a period when many middle-aged couples realize that they have neglected close friendships, the focus having been on relatedness within the family or between the marital partners (Lowenthal et al., 1975). The neglect of friendships in this particular era no doubt contributes to the sense of loneliness and isolation experienced by many who have lost a mate through death or divorce in the mid-life period.

Psychodynamic Theories of Adult Development

Psychodynamic theories of human development vary in the extent to which they address the strains and challenges of the middle years. Within the Freudian framework, adult development issues are part of a deterministic scheme where conflicts and strains of the oedipal period are reworked at each later crisis point. Typical mid-life crisis events such as extramarital acting out would be understood in terms of an individual's attempt to deal with parental figures of an earlier developmental era. Incestuous wishes might be replayed in the choice of younger partners. Similarly, struggles with a boss or superior, the wish to become free and independent, in Levinson's terms "one's own man" (1974) can all be interpreted in terms of the oedipal rivalry with an all-powerful father.

Kubie, in addressing himself to the activity/passivity changes in men and women in the middle years, conceptualizes this phenomenon in reductionistic terms as well: "The drive to become both sexes has pre-genital, phallic, genital, and oedipal ingredients; it becomes reactivated repeatedly in the latency period, in puberty, in adolescence, in adult life and again in various stages of the aging process" (1974, p. 409).

Jung (1954) is explicit in suggesting that psychological events of adulthood cannot be reduced simply to a repetition of oedipal conflicts. According to Jung, adult life or middle adulthood is the time of optimum personality development. In middle adulthood the individual is free to develop those sides of himself which he has had to repress until now. In contrast to Kubie, who conceptualizes the shift in activity/passivity as essentially a neurotic event, Jung suggests that this shift is not only adaptive but enriching as well. Tender and more nurturant aspects of the male had to be kept out of awareness in order to carry out socially expected tasks which required assertiveness and aggressiveness. Women, on the other hand, had to be the caretakers and comfort givers and therefore could allow their nurturant tendencies full expression while having to restrain their strivings for self-assertion and independence. Much as one might question, particularly today, whether this reciprocal arrangement is not mainly due to cultural factors, some of the recent life cycle research data tend to support Jung's conceptual scheme.

Jung also focuses on the second major issue of the middle years, i.e., on the beginning confrontation with one's own mortality and finiteness. Again Jung differs from Freud who in *Thoughts on War and Death* rules out the possibility that man can genuinely acknowledge the possibility of his own mortality: "Attitude toward death is far from straightforward. We were of course prepared to maintain that death was a necessary outcome of life . . . that death was natural, undeniable and unavoidable. In reality, however, we were accustomed to behave as if it were otherwise . . . our own death is indeed unimaginable, and whenever we make an attempt to imagine it we can perceive that we really survive as spectators. Hence the psychoanalytic school would venture upon the assertion that at bottom no one believes in his own death, or to put the same thing another way, in the unconscious everyone is convinced of his own immortality" (1959, p. 304).

It is precisely the necessity of giving up one's fantasies of immortality, omnipotence and grandiosity that is seen by contemporary analysts as representing the major psychological task of the middle years. Marmor describes the psychological experience of those years as consisting of ". . . loss of one's youthful self-image, the increased frequency of illness and death among relatives and friends, and loss of children who leave home, and the loss of love in the 'tired' marriage . . . most significantly, however, the loss of phantasy hopes of youth and an inescapable confrontation with the fact of mortality represent the most recurring stresses of mid-life" (1974, p. 73).

Jacques (1965) describes mid-life as that period when the individual is forced to come to terms with his grandiose omnipotence. He has to give up his magical dependence on the good object and instead develop a capacity to tolerate his own shortcomings and destructiveness. Jacques' formulation, though in object relation terms, closely resembles those of Erikson and Gould.

Erikson sees the middle years as years of moving from the stage of generativity to the stage of integrity, as involving an increasing ability to accept "one's own and only life cycle and the people who have become significant to it as something that had to be and that, by necessity, permitted of no substitutions. It thus means a new, different love of one's parents, free of the wish that they should be different and an acceptance of the fact one's life is one's own responsibility" (1959, p. 98). In Erikson's view, the middle years involve acknowledgment of mortality as well as an assessment of remaining options, options that include caring beyond the narrow bonds of family.

Similar issues are addressed by Cath (1962), who describes the transition from creator and doer in the middle years to progenitor and observer and the effects of this shift on the marital and family relationships. Klein (1963), on the other hand, suggests that adjustment to aging will to a large extent depend on the extent to which the individual has resolved issues of envy and rivalry. Being able to watch others and specifically one's children grow up without undue competition and envy enables one to identify with the satisfactions of youth without having to spoil one's own satisfaction by envy or malcontent.

Kernberg (1977) in discussing *Pathological Narcissism in Middle Age* suggests the following life tasks as central in the middle years: shift in perspective to include the entire life span; reversal in external and internal rates of change; acknowledgment of limits of one's creativity; the issue of ego identity within the time perspective, i.e., the individual's ability to acknowledge and accept characterological limitations and the issues of loss, mourning and death.

Roger Gould's (1977) definition of the mid-life task involves two essential components: (a) Adulthood consists of increasingly refined and evolving changes in self-definition which create conflicts and anxiety because of old prohibitions and rules which were part and parcel of a childhood frame of reference; and (b) adulthood requires a universal developmental task that accompanies the developing self-definitions. This task involves the relinquishing of what Gould calls the "illusion of absolute safety." This illusion of absolute safety would seem to be a vestige of infantile omnipotence, involving insistence on the possibilities of magical solutions and the accompanying notion that separation and individuation can be avoided.

To some extent, the issues and the research data summarized in the preceding section tend to support the emphasis on loss, giving up of options and general retrenchment of the mid-life years suggested by various psychodynamic theories. Research on the whole has not addressed itself to the possibility of options and gains in the middle years. It therefore lends support to the popular notion of mid-life crisis. Nevertheless, the term crisis refers to both danger and opportunity and therefore merely denotes a change in course and not a harbinger of catastrophe. Vaillant's (1977) study of successful men is an exception to the crisis orientation of mid-life research in that it demonstrates that the phenomenological experience of being middle-aged can be one of satisfaction and pleasure provided one has been able to adopt increasingly mature ways—Vaillant refers to the maturing of ego defenses—to cope with the strains of living. What needs to be challenged by future research is the notion that giving up one's grandiose fantasies can only be painful. The process of relinquishing something is indeed painful; however, mastering and resolving a conflict can have its own inherent satisfactions as well as potential promises. The latter is suggested in the changing nature of relatedness and intimacy in middle adulthood referred to in a number of studies. (Lionells and Mann, 1978; Lowenthal and Weiss, 1975).

Implications of Mid-Life Changes for the Couple and the Family

Theory and research each have their own level of abstraction. They need to be translated in terms of direct applicability to family and marital issues. Furthermore, some attention will have to be given to cultural factors that perhaps may appear developmental in nature, and to the interactions between developmental and sociocultural factors.

There is little question that the early 40s are indeed a time of stress and tension for married couples. Accident proneness increases; alcoholism is on the rise; stress symptoms such as coronary problems or high blood pressure are on the increase (Rogers, 1973).

Most men in their middle adult years view the middle years as a time of having it made, when they can finally relax and enjoy the fruits of their strivings. On the other hand, today's middle-aged women anticipate their middle years somewhat differently. Rather than anticipating "having it made," the middle-aged woman looks to the ensuing years as full of activity and increasing freedom to pursue her own interests. This has brought new challenges, demands, and conflicts for the woman as well as the family. For instance, as noted by Notman in Chapter 6 of this volume, when a woman who has been the central family caretaker makes a serious work commitment, typical family interaction patterns are upset and family stability can be threatened.

Confronted with the actuality of the middle years, neither men nor women seem to be particularly satisfied or at ease with themselves or each other. For the man, job satisfactions are not as great as anticipated. The wish to start afresh is experienced and at times acted upon. Verbalizations of dissatisfaction and of the wish to make a complete change often arouse considerable anxiety in his spouse, who perhaps for the first time in many years sees a possibility for working towards her own satisfactions. She would like to enjoy some of the job security benefits in order to pursue her own interests. Exploration and pursuit of independent interests on the part of the woman come at a time when the man is experiencing an increased need for support and nurturance from her.

Diverging adaptations for the middle-aged couple are perhaps most evident in the sexual area. For the man in his 40s and 50s, sexual pleasure becomes a changing experience. In earlier years, sexual drive was reflected in frequency of orgasm, ease of erection, intense and forceful ejaculation and a relatively short refractory period. In the 40s, there is often a gradual lessening of the frequency of orgasm; sexual pleasure is less exclusively related to genitally localized sensations and becomes more sensuous. Prolonged and more intense stimulation is needed for erection to take place.

The man's reaction to these changes depends largely on how secure he is within himself, to what extent his self-esteem is sexualized in machismo fashion and whether he can begin to acknowledge his own needs for tenderness which are emerging as part of the aging process.

While the man experiences some slowing down of sexual response, the woman in her middle years often becomes sexually more responsive (Gadpaille, 1975; Kaplan, 1974). She experiences a sense of liberation and a thrust towards increased activity (Brooks, 1975) that transcends the area of sexuality. Women in the middle years are becoming increasingly aware of their competence and often wish to move out of the circumscribed social and familial roles of motherhood. This movement towards increased self-assertiveness goes hand in hand with the more freely experienced interest in sexual activity. Sexual and generalized assertiveness on the woman's part becomes a difficult challenge to her middle-aged mate who experiences uncertainty regarding his potency.

Given a changed attitude towards and freedom with sexuality, the woman entering menopause may never experience the problems so often considered typical of the cessation of menses. Nevertheless, middle age still looms as a threat to the woman who experiences an upsurge of sexual feelings but is hampered either by sociocultural stereotypes or by her own narcissistic needs. The woman who has had little satisfaction other than her narcissistic investment in her children will experience middle age with the spectre of menopause as a serious blow to her self-esteem. If she feels compelled to maintain a youthful self-image, she will experience further distress and envy as she is confronted with the emerging sexuality and attractiveness of an adolescent child. Depression, irritability, avoidance of sexuality or the converse, flight into extramarital affairs, may be the result of the middle-aged woman's dilemma. She, too, particularly at mid-life, needs the support, reassurance, and sexual attention of her partner. However, in many instances she not only puts distance between herself and her partner, but she also interprets his greater sexual uncertainty at mid-life as an active act of rejection. In short, interacting anxieties of the partners can turn possible rejection into a self-fulfilling prophecy.

Changing sexuality and level of assertiveness are only part of the source of conflict often encountered in middle-aged couples. Today's middle-aged woman experiences a push towards self-assertion not only because of intrapsychic changes, but also because of the cultural impact of the women's liberation movement. Even if she has combined her need for independence and a measure of separateness with some degree of support and nurturance for her spouse, she frequently takes up the cudgel for activism to an extreme degree. Experiencing little understanding of her partner's dependent needs, she, in effect, demands repayment for imagined or real past transgressions on her rights as a woman. The often rigid acceptance of the stance of the liberated woman presents today's middle-aged husband with increasing threats and conflicts. At the time where he might even be open to essentially "equal rights" within the marriage, he is frequently intimidated and exasperated by his wife's insistence on a role reversal rather than an equalization of the relationship.

Besides the strains arising from intrapsychic and interpersonal conflicts in the middle years, additional stress is related to intergenerational issues. The empty nest syndrome represents both a challenge and an opportunity. For the first time in some 20 years, the couple is relatively alone without the continued presence of a third individual. In many instances, the 20 years of child rearing have indeed separated husband and wife to such a degree that they have become strangers. The reality of being alone with one another may reveal the fact that neither partner is able to relate intimately to the other and that, at best, they can live alongside one another now that they lack the common focus of child rearing.

Growing children further represent tensions in terms of the comparisons they encourage with times past. Middle-aged parents who have not come to terms with the limitations they need to confront because of their age and who are locked into a narcissistic character structure will find it difficult to view their growing children with feelings that are free of envy and competition. Kernberg states that the middle-aged patient with narcissistic pathology has "particular difficulties in facing the growing independence of adolescent children. To empathize with this growing world of adolescence while feeling subtly and increasingly excluded from it requires maturity, empathy with others that compensates for the natural sense of loss and mourning, overcoming or neutralization of the universal feeling of envy" (Kernberg, 1977, p. 20). Feelings of envy and competition, though particularly prevalent when one is dealing with pathological narcissism, are certainly part and parcel of the normal adult experience of seeing one's children grow up and experience what to many parents seem like unlimited possibilities and freedom from responsibilities.

Given the emphasis on loss, mourning of opportunities no longer available, competition with and envy of younger individuals and the general sense of being "over the hill," are there gains and options in the middle years as Erikson suggests? Do these gains present simply a denial rather than an accurate reflection of the nature of the midlife experience for men and women?

A pilot study of age-related countertransference attitudes (Lionells and Mann, 1978) indicates that the middle years are characterized by a movement towards greater interiority and greater individuation, a movement which is related to changes in the sense of self. The younger middle-aged individual sees himself in relation to others around him; he thinks in relational terms where satisfactions and security are intricately linked to and supplied by the other person in one's life. Older individuals, who have gone beyond the middle years, on the other hand focus more on a sense of themselves;

they seem to have arrived at a sense of their own identity that is relatively independent of the reflected appraisals of others. The older individual views his relatedness to others in a way that involves less symbiosis and allows for more individuation, and separateness. In concrete terms, this seems to indicate that having passed the early 40s, there is the possibility of a different kind of relatedness. Each partner feels freer to pursue what he or she needs in terms of a sense of self-fulfillment and accomplishment; at the same time, the partners can be available for one another with lessened competitiveness and rivalry; they can respect one another's wish for separateness but also have interdependence and mutuality.

Clinical Implications of Mid-Life Issues and Options

Misconceptions regarding the middle years of life are widespread and most clinicians are affected by the cultural stereotypes regarding aging. A study of therapists carried out under the auspices of the William Alanson White Institute found that therapists differ along age lines in their assessment of issues and options confronted by middle-aged patients. The possibility that the middle years can be growth-producing despite some losses was acknowledged only by those therapists who were themselves past the middle years. Furthermore, younger analysts focused on different issues with their middle-aged patients than did older therapists. Younger therapists stressed issues of the patient in his marriage and the nature of the relationship. They were very much aware of the narcissistic injuries inflicted by aging; they mentioned issues such as physical attractiveness, health, status and career, issues that were usually mentioned within a competitive context. In other words, the emphasis was on comparisons with younger individuals. Younger therapists felt that adult life presented an increasing constriction of potential coupled with a concomitant turning towards one's partner for expanding life satisfactions. They exhibited a certain amount of cynicism about mid-life. Senior therapists, i.e., those past 60 years, were more concerned with the self-determining individual. They defined mid-life and mid-life crisis in terms of an individual's experience of himself and talked about middle adulthood as a time for self-examination and mastery. Senior therapists' overall view of the middle years was couched in terms of the growing differentiation of the adult individual and the vicissitudes of that individuation. To the older clinician, the middle years seem to provide a new stage in the life cycle where the person begins to define him or herself not only in contrast to his parents, but also in contrast to his spouse, his family and his children. The older therapists felt that the middle years represent an opportunity to turn back from involvement while promoting a new freedom to participate in relationships as an independent, self-sufficient individual who finds fulfillment in his or her own life.

An understanding of these differing assessments of the middle years depending on the age of the therapist would seem to be essential in working with the middle-aged patient, since it will help to minimize countertransference distortions that can affect the therapeutic process.

Besides age-specific countertransference reactions, work with middle-aged individuals in crisis also needs to take into account age-related transference reactions. The middle-aged patient who comes for treatment may be particularly anxious with a therapist considerably younger than himself. The younger therapist is seen by the middle-aged patient as someone who is not really capable of supplying support; in addition, feelings of competitiveness and envy may reach such intensity that the patient unconsciously needs to destroy the therapist and render him impotent. Although envy at any point has a distinctly destructive potential, envy stemming from middle-aged narcissism and directed at a younger therapist can become a major obstacle in therapy.

In addition to transference/countertransference issues related to the respective chronological ages of therapist and patient, the middle-aged patient presents some age-related issues in terms of expectations from therapy. For one, the middle-aged patient beginning therapy frequently has some very specific goals in terms of what he or she wants to accomplish and the time required to reach these goals. The middle-aged individual coming for therapy is, on some level, aware of the limited time left. The insistence on some time commitment on the part of the therapist regarding duration of treatment is not just an expression of a neurotic effort to control.

Similarly, the middle-aged patient tends to establish a working alliance with the therapist that is less often characterized by dependence and regression; instead, there is often a definite attempt to relate to the therapist as an equal. In short, age factors shape both context and content of therapy as well as transference and counter-transference attitudes. Before labeling a particular middle-aged patient as resistive, distant or inappropriately controlling, therapists working with middle-aged individuals and couples have to assess the extent to which a patient's behavior and symptomatology are age-related and to what extent the therapist may be blinded by his own chronological age.

Two clinical examples might help to illustrate some of the issues with which middle-aged couples deal and also the extent to which given difficulties are specifically age-related or derivatives of earlier neurotic adaptations.

A middle-aged couple came for treatment because of problems related to day-to-day responsibilities for elderly parents, problems that threatened to disrupt the couple's marriage. The couple was at the typical mid-life juncture: He was a successful executive; she was returning to school for an advanced degree. The elderly parents were in their own right successful and until recently independent; now in their 80s, they were becoming increasingly frail, forgetful and no longer able to care for themselves adequately or safely. The middle-aged son found it impossible to cope with the changed requirements of the relationship. He needed to be firm, in making some decision for his parents that would affect their style of living. Instead of being able to take assertive action, he demanded that his wife take care of his parents since "that way they would not get angry."

In the course of therapy, it became evident that this man had never truly separated from his parents, still was in terror of his father and needed to be the "good child" as he had always been. Only when this stance began to interfere with his own marriage —his wife had become increasingly depressed and angry at having to take care of her in-laws—was he ready to work through some of his earlier feelings and get in touch with his rage. He had been acting out the latter since his seemingly benign concern for his parents with its lack of supervision increasingly exposed them to accidents and danger.

In this particular example intergenerational issues, never resolved in adolescence and young adulthood, clearly became reactivated in the middle years. Most middle-aged adults seem to be able to deal with their parents' advancing age with somewhat less conflict. On the other hand, quite often unresolved familial conflicts make their appearance in settings other than the immediate family, and difficulties in relation to a boss, teacher, older colleague, or mentor may really be expressions of childhood conflicts.

While the foregoing example is one where separation and individuation issues began to interfere with adult adjustment, the following example represents one where differentiation between neurotic strivings and age-appropriate issues proved to be of importance.

An outwardly successful man in his late 40s was experiencing increasing tension, dissatisfaction and depression. He had rapidly risen in his work; his personal life had been fulfilling and his children seemed to negotiate their adolescence without undue conflict. Gradually, however, the marriage had begun to deteriorate. Strains in the marriage seemed to coincide with the husband's wish to make a total change and "start from scratch." His wife, at this particular time, was looking forward to her own return to school so that she too could embark on a career. Anger in response to her husband's threatened decision to quit his job thinly masked her anxiety over apparently being deprived of her chance to enter the professional world.

Therapy helped this man to sort out and evaluate his varying options and to discard those that were neurotically motivated. In essence he was able to differentiate between age-appropriate dissatisfaction and unresolved childhood conflicts. Although the wish for change was largely non-neurotic, the impulse to throw away past professional gains was an attempt to act out an underlying grandiosity. In dreams and fantasies this man expected that his "newly chosen" profession would lead to instant, worldwide recognition. Relinquishing an expectation which would require another lifetime to become reality enabled the patient to pursue a more clearly adaptive course of action.

SUMMARY

The mid-life years put age-specific strains on couples and families. Parents in middle age often go through a crisis period which reflects the impact of becoming middle-aged. The impact of the middle years is related to changes in passivity/activity in both men and women and to the increasing realization of one's finiteness and potential mortality. Much of the acting out in this time of life has to do with attempts to deny the realities of aging. However, putting stress only on the crisis aspects of the middle years is to neglect some of the options that are also associated with mid-life, options that arise out of a changed sense of self which allows both greater individuation and more intimate relatedness than before.

Clinical work with middle-aged couples and families also needs to take into account the diverging adaptations of men and women in mid-life. The role of envy and competition often experienced by the middle-aged parent of a growing child should not be overlooked.

In addition, therapists working with mid-life patients need to be aware of their own attitudes towards the middle years since they color the assessment of therapeutic goals.

Theory and research have addressed themselves mainly to the crises aspects of the middle years. The challenges and options of mid-life, particularly as they refer to the nature of interpersonal relatedness in middle adulthood, are less clearly understood or delineated in the professional literature. Erikson (1959), Lowenthal et al. (1975), Mann (1977a, b) and Vaillant (1977) suggest that middle adulthood brings with it not only crises and challenges but options as well. These options seem to refer to changes in the direction of self-fulfillment, to a different sense of self and to a different kind of relatedness to oneself and to others. Further clarification of these options will have to await future research.

REFERENCES

American Heritage Dictionary. New York: Dell, 1977.

BACK, K.: Transition to aging and self-aging. *International Journal of Aging and Human Development,* 1971, 2:296-304.

BROOKS, B.: Developmental aspects of aging in women. *Archives of General Psychiatry,* 1975, 32.

BROWN, T.: *The Middle-Life Search for Vocation.* Paper presented at the American Personnel and Guidance Association Meeting, Chicago, Ill., March 1972.

CATH, S.: Grief, loss and educational disorders in the aging process. In M. A. Berezin and S. Cath (Eds.), *Geriatric Psychiatry.* New York: International Universities Press, 1962.

CLAUSEN, J.: The life course of individuals. In M. Riley, M. Johnson and A. Fones (Eds.), *Aging and Society: A Sociological View of the Life Course,* Vol. 3. New York: Russell Sage, 1972.

Cox, R. D.: *Stress Adaptation and Growth in the Adult Years: An Explanation of Normative Development.* Paper presented at the Annual Friends Hospital Conference, Philadelphia, October 1976.

Erikson, E.: Identity and the life cycle. *Psychological Issues,* 1959, 1:50-100.

Farrell, M.: Abstract. *Behavior Today,* March, 1975.

Freud, S.: Thoughts on War and Death. *Collected Papers,* Vol. 4. New York: Basic Books, 1959.

Gadpaille, W. J.: *The Cycles of Sex.* New York: Charles Scribner's Sons, 1975.

Gould, R. L.: The phases of adult life: A study of developmental psychology. *American Journal of Psychiatry,* 1972, 129:521-531.

Gould, R. L.: *Psychoanalytically Based Theory of Adult Development.* Paper presented at Annual Friends Hospital Conference, Philadelphia, Pa., October 1977.

Havighurst, R. J.: History of developmental psychology: Socialization and personality development through the life span. In P. B. Baltes and K. W. Schaie (Eds.), *Life-span Developmental Psychology: Personality and Socialization.* New York: Academic Press, 1973.

Jacques, E.: Death and the mid-life crisis. *International Journal of Psychoanalysis,* 1965, 46:502-514.

Jung, C. J.: *The Development of Personality.* New York: Pantheon Books, Inc., 1954.

Kaplan, H. S.: *The New Sex Therapy.* New York: Brunner/Mazel, 1974.

Kernberg, O. F.: *Pathological Narcissism in Middle Age.* Paper presented at the Baylor College of Medicine, Houston, Texas, November 1977.

Kimmel, D. C.: *Adulthood and Aging.* New York: John Wiley & Sons, Inc., 1974.

Klein, M.: *Our Adult World.* New York: Basic Books, 1963.

Kubie, L. S.: The drive to become both sexes. *The Psychoanalytic Quarterly,* 1974, 43: 349-426.

Levenson, E. A.: Changing concepts of intimacy in psychoanalytic practice. *Journal of Contemporary Psychoanalysis,* 1974, 10:359-369.

Levinson, D., Darrow, C., Klein, E., Levinson, M., & McKee, B.: Men in early adulthood and the mid-life transition. In D. F. Ricks, A. Thomas, and M. Roff (Eds.), *Life History Research in Psychopathology,* Vol. 3. Minneapolis: University of Minnesota Press, 1974.

Lionells, M. & Mann, C. H.: Patterns of mid-life in transition. In G. D. Goldman and D. S. Milman (Eds.), *Man and Woman in Transition.* Dubuque, Iowa: Kendall-Hunt Co., 1978.

Lowenthal, M. E. & Chiriboga, D.: Transition to the empty nest: Crisis, challenge or relief? *Archives of General Psychiatry,* 1972, 26:8-14.

Lowenthal, M., Thurnher, M., & Chiriboga, D.: *Four Stages of Life.* San Francisco: Jossey-Bass, 1975.

Lowenthal, M. E. & Weiss, L.: Intimacy and crises in adulthood. In E. Schlossberg and B. Entine (Eds.), *Counselling Adults.* Monterey, California: Brooks/Cole, 1975.

Mann, C. H.: *The Changing Nature of Human Relatedness and Intimacy in Middle Adulthood.* Paper presented at the Sixth International Forum for Psychoanalysis, Berlin, Germany, August 1977 (a).

Mann, C. H.: *Mid-life Issues—the Dynamics of Mid-life Changes.* Paper presented at Annual Friends Hospital Conference, Philadelphia, Pa., October 1977 (b).

Marmor, J.: *Psychiatry in Transition.* New York: Brunner/Mazel, 1974.

Neugarten, B.: Continuities and discontinuities of psychological issues into adult life. *Human Development,* 1969, 12:121-130.

Rogers, K.: *Mid-career Crisis.* Paper presented at the William Alanson White Institute, 1973.

Schecter, D. & Lippman, P.: *The Study of the Human Life Cycle: Patterns of Attach-*

ment (Symbiosis, Fusion) vs. Separation (Individuation) with Particular Emphasis on Adult Development. Paper presented at the Fifth International Forum of Psychoanalysis, Zurich, 1974.

SCHLOSSBERG, N. K.: Adults in transition. *ERIC Microfiche,* 1966, ED01696.

SHEEHY, G. *Passages.* New York: N. P. Dutton & Co., 1976.

SODDY, K. & KIDSON, M.: *Men in Middle Life.* London: Lippincott Co., 1967.

TERKEL, L.: *Working.* New York: Partheon, 1974.

VAILLANT, G. E.: *Adaptation to Life.* Boston: Little, Brown & Co., 1977.

Chapter 9

Divorce in Mid-Life: Clinical Implications and Applications

Nathan W. Turner

INTRODUCTION

Current literature by Sheehy (1976), Vaillant (1977), Gould (1978), Glick (1975), Neugarten (1968), Lidz (1968), and others documents the variety of life events, such as stagnation or advancement in career, biological/physiological deficits, aging parents, marriage reassessment, and economic pressures that not only challenge but provide the occasion for growth and/or decline in the middle years. One challenge often confronted in mid-life involves the handling of disenchantment with the marital relationship and the possibility of separation or divorce.

Marital disenchantment and decisions to separate or divorce are seen as the product of multiple determinants which include: unmet expectations in the marriage, rewards/costs in marriage, children, in-laws, money, unarticulated changes in one's life circumstances and styles of coping with life stress. Furthermore, as Glick (1975) and Norton and Glick (1976) point out, there are changes occurring in our culture that also have a major impact on the traditional marriage. Some of these changes include a greater social acceptance of divorce as a means of resolving marital problems, increasing acceptance of serial monogamy as a valid alternative to traditional marriage, and an increasing awareness of the discrepancy between traditional sex roles and the culture's current emphasis on companionship and equality within the relationship.

In order to understand some of the complexities and vicissitudes experienced by the couple confronted with marital disenchantment, a comprehensive view of the total process, commencing with estrangement and concluding with the post-divorce series of adjustments, will be presented. The chapter is organized into three parts. First is an abbreviated and highly selective review of several theoretical models in the literature of separation and divorce. The second is a presentation of a comprehensive model of separation and divorce counseling, integrating various models of divorce with the decision-making model presented by Janis and Mann (1977). The third part considers the clinical implications for assessment and potential treatment applications derived from the model.

THEORETICAL BACKGROUND

They are symbiotically attached people who are terrified of being alone, of being individuals in their own right. They are unable to problem solve within the marriage, nor are they capable of leaving the marriage and problem solving free of the torturing mate. They have low self-esteem and accept being treated without respect by their mates rather than being alone (Martin, 1976, pp. 171-172).

The emotional dependence described above is typical of the dynamics involved in marriage and/or divorce counseling. The study of divorce and divorce counseling is relatively new in comparison to other fields of behavioral science investigation (Freund, 1974). The negative value traditionally associated with divorce is becoming more neutral; evidence of this change can be seen in books such as *Creative Divorce* (Krantzler, 1975) and *The Courage to Divorce* (Gettleman & Markowitz, 1975), which challenge the reader to consider the positive values in separation and divorce.

An increase in alternative life-styles and living arrangements by individuals of all ages, including the middle-aged population, serves as a clue that change is occurring both within and outside of the American marriage.* "There seems little doubt that a basic transformation of the institution of marriage is under way and that many variables are influencing the direction of the change" (Norton and Glick, 1976, p. 17). New rules and contracts for marriage may allow expectations for relationships, including marriage, to merge with the de facto conditions of our society.

The act and experience of divorce serve as a continual challenge to the conventional wisdom regarding the social institution we call marriage. In spite of this, we continue to view marriage in a romantic, idealistic manner, with the assumption that marriage is for life. The social distortion in the variety of social myths held about marriage arises from assumptions about marriage. A transformation of marriage is occurring as a result of multiple variables influencing the future of marriage (Bernard, 1972).

The divorce process is characterized by both grief and growth, rejection of the lost love object, and acceptance of new patterns of life. In developing a theoretical framework for divorce, it is important to establish a comprehensive view of the total process, commencing with estrangement (Goode, 1956; Levinger, 1976; McCall and Simmons, 1966) and concluding with the post-divorce series of adjustments.

Prior to actual separation or divorce, various small acts serve to create alienation, coolness, indifference, and gradual erosion of the meaning in the relationship. The small, daily, often-forgotten decisions to avoid, resist, or discount one's spouse inaugurate a process which may lead to separation or divorce. At the other end of the continuum, one encounters a post-divorce series of adjustments in dealing with in-laws, children's needs and rights, changes in

---

* There is no divorce boom in middle age; there are more divorces at mid-life today only because there are more divorces at every age today (Hunt and Hunt, 1977). Approximately half of all divorces occur in the first seven years of the marriage. Clearly, the divorce rate declines with age. Only about 12 percent of divorcing males are 40 or over and about 14 percent of divorcing females are 45 or older.

economic status, changes in occupation and social status, potential continuing changes in relating to the former spouse, and potential new, intimate relationships for oneself and for one's former spouse.

Wiseman (1975) has developed a theory for the process and crisis of divorce composed of five overlapping stages, based on the Kübler-Ross grief model: 1) denial, 2) loss and depression, 3) anger and ambivalence, 4) reorientation of life-style and identity, and 5) acceptance and integration. Because of the newness of the field, theoretical development of models for divorce counseling has been slow (Fisher, 1975). However, several models have been suggested. Smart (1977) has provided a major contribution to theory development by applying Erikson's eight-stage developmental model to the stages of divorce process. Bohannan (1970), on the other hand, distinguished six experiences during the divorce process which may vary in order and/or overlap:

1) Emotional divorce begins when the spouses withhold emotion from their relationship. It generally begins before separation and continues for some time afterward.
2) Legal divorce occurs when the final decree is handed down by the judge.
3) Economic divorce occurs when the individuals set up separate housekeeping and separate their belongings.
4) Coparental divorce is the separation of mothering and fathering roles that is made necessary when separate residences are established.
5) Community divorce involves the loosening of bonds with some old friends and acquaintances, and the beginning of new relationships.
6) Psychic divorce deals with individual autonomy. Persons who have lived together for years must separate their identities when they divorce.

In contrast to both Smart and Bohannan, Weiss (1975) cites three major stages of divorce:

1) Erosion of love and persistence of attachment; focus is on the ambivalence that surrounds the breaking of love bonds.
2) Separation brings feelings of distress, euphoria, and loneli-

ness, and necessitates identity changes that correspond to
Bohannan's psychic divorce.

3) Starting over includes three substages: (a) shock and denial;
(b) transition (i.e., disorganization, depression, and unman-
ageable restlessness) ; and (c) recovery, which usually takes
two to four years to complete.

Although most models of divorce counseling focus on the separation, divorce, and post-divorce processes (Bohannan, 1970; Smart,
1977; Wiseman, 1975), it is important to consider antecedent processes and behaviors as well (Bjorksten, 1974). Antecedent behaviors
and events can serve as precipitating factors for later relationship
difficulties. An example of this process is provided by a female client
who presented with a desire to divorce her husband, feeling that the
marriage of two and a half years was over for her. It was a first marriage for both and they had no children. Upon careful investigation,
it became clear that she had entered the marriage with a conscious
desire to "change" her husband-to-be in several significant ways. Her
secret wish had never been shared with him. After two and a half
years when he did not change, she became angry with him, felt disenchanted, and wanted out of the marriage.

Decision-making theory and research (Janis and Mann, 1977)
are especially relevant in an analysis of the separation and divorce
process. The implications of decisions pertaining to separation and/
or divorce are the particular emphasis of the model for divorce counseling proposed in this chapter. Special importance is attached to
antecedent decisions which result in relationship disenchantment.
The following stages represent a comprehensive model for divorce
counseling, integrating various other models, theories, and research
findings.

RELATIONSHIP DISENCHANTMENT

Disenchantment is based on the psychological violation of largely
known but unverbalized contracts (Sager, 1976). The present model
explicates six sources of relationship disenchantment.

Growth or Change in Self or Spouse: Growth or change in either
person in the relationship often serves to trigger dormant needs or
dynamics within the marital/relationship dyad. With the advent of

the feminist movement (human rights), some women have begun to claim their need to individuate as persons beyond the prescribed roles of wife and mother. Major changes in traditional sex roles within the American home are occurring (Bernard, 1972; Reed, 1976). Reactions of the men involved have ranged from being threatened to acceptance and outright support. When one partner grows and changes, the other partner is forced to react to the change in some manner. Such forced reactions are often accompanied initially by the pain of disenchantment with the idealized spouse image (Brown, 1976).

Impact of Major Life Events: Major life events can also initiate relationship disenchantment when one partner changes in reaction to such events. The trauma of physical injury, unexpected illness, loss of a job or career, onset of emotional illness, or substantial change in values and life orientation can initiate emotional reactions in one spouse, to which the other spouse reacts. When such life events impact to force behavioral change upon one or both partners, disenchantment and resentment can begin. Abrupt role changes, for which the partners have not contracted, may not be received happily by the other person, who may be pressured into more of a nurturant, supportive role than is tolerable (Sager, 1976). Likewise, major life events may precipitate a marriage. The death of a parent, for instance, may serve as an antecedent event to "set up" a marriage soon after the death, in order to meet dependency needs which are no longer met by the deceased parent.

Social Comparisons: As a marriage develops, both spouses are bound to make various social comparisons of their marriage with the marriages of their acquaintances. These silent, and occasionally verbal, comparisons may result in unfavorable judgments about one's marriage. Such negative judgments are usually directed at one's spouse, who is found deficient—especially in mid-life when sufficient years have been logged in to make a rather solid comparison—and disenchantment develops.

Shift in Rewards/Costs in the Marriage: When one spouse makes a shift in her/his view of the rewards versus the emotional or physical costs of the relationship, the resulting feelings may be the beginnings of disenchantment.

A dual-professional, childless couple in their early 30s sought marital counseling with typical presenting problems: poor communication, a dissatisfying sexual relationship, and disagreement over whether to purchase a first home. Underlying the presenting problems, however, were the wife's unrecognized dependency needs. Her unconscious security needs led her to demand that her husband change his vocation and double his income within six months, or she would divorce him. Earlier in the marriage, the wife had viewed their relationship as a highly successful dual marriage. As time went on, however, she became disenchanted with her husband's degree of career success, which was less than her own. When she feared that she might become the primary wage earner in the marriage, she shifted her view of the rewards in the marriage, feeling that the emotional and economic costs were greater than she could tolerate. Her shift triggered relationship disenchantment, a separation and divorce.

Third Party Attraction/Attachment: Attraction and emotional attachment to a third party represent another possible impetus for emotional disenchantment with one's partner. When one's spouse begins to "look around" at the opposite sex in a serious manner, it can be symptomatic of relationship unrest for a variety of reasons. Jealousy can result and can be the source of further tension within the relationship. Clinically, attraction to a third party can be interpreted as a symptom of marital problems or as a sign of individual health in moving out of an unhealthy marital relationship (Lieberman, 1976). Individual growth and change in one partner may result in attraction to a third party if the other marital partner fails to respond to the growth in a positive, supportive, and accepting manner.

Beginning of Gradual Withdrawal/Disenchantment: Gradual withdrawal of one partner from the other can be slow and subtle. A small change in routine, habit, or style may be an initial sign of disenchantment. Changes in personal grooming and hygiene or patterns of work (including time spent at work) may be symptomatic of the withdrawal. Often the decision to begin withdrawal may be an unconscious one, since to "own" the decision consciously would be too painful to accept immediately. Consequently, questions like "What's wrong with you?" or "You don't seem like yourself lately!" are given vague, ineffectual answers by the spouse, who may not know consciously why she/he actually feels the way she/he does. Individuals in such situations may feel like withdrawing, yet deny the feeling. Nevertheless, the beginning of withdrawal is a major sign of the beginnings of relationship disenchantment.

DECISIONAL CONFLICT: STRESS, AMBIVALENCE, CONFLICT

Both the decision to marry and the decision to separate or divorce can result in intense intrapsychic conflict. Symptoms of the decisional conflict may include questions such as "Should I or shouldn't I?", "Will it last?", "Is this the right person for me?", "Is it over?", "Will I hurt my spouse?", or "Is there any way to correct our problems and keep the relationship going?" Discussed below are three potential conflict areas that are common in decisions to marry, separate and/or divorce.

Surfacing of Opposing Pulls: Janis and Mann (1977) have developed the concept of "decisional conflict" to describe the situation in which an individual feels opposing decisions pulling her/him in different directions (e.g., "Should I stay in the marriage or leave it?"). Common symptoms of decisional conflict include vacillation, hesitation, feelings of uncertainty, and acute signs of emotional stress. One source of stress in decisional conflict is the feeling that one is risking major loss in whatever decision is considered. The intensity of the resulting stress symptoms depends upon the perceived magnitude of the losses the person anticipates from any of the decisions she/he may make. Common symptoms of stress in making such difficult decisions include a desire to escape, self-blame, and feelings of apprehensiveness (Janis and Mann, 1977). These symptoms of stress are common among clients in separation and divorce counseling.

Ambivalence and Double Binds: The decision to separate from or divorce one's partner usually is filled with ambivalence. To see and feel the good as well as the bad in one's relationship is to experience this ambivalence. The double bind involved in a decision regarding the continuation of the marriage is the feeling that "I'll lose if I stay in the marriage and I'll lose if I leave the marriage!"

The more ambivalent one feels and the more one senses that she/he is in a double bind, the greater the chances of disenchantment. Ambivalence and double bind feelings serve as barriers to effective decision-making. Perceived double binds need to be assessed clinically to determine whether the binds have a basis in fact or are self-imposed through distorted perceptions of reality.

Conflict—To Decide or Not to Decide: Decisional conflict begins as a stress reaction to the opposing pulls involved in making a decision about separation or divorce. Following the initial period of stress comes a period of ambivalence and feelings of being in a double bind. Finally, the internal conflict becomes apparent to the individual and a key question is "Whether I will decide or not decide to remain in the marriage?" It is important to note, however, that a decision to "not decide" is also a clear decision. The decisional conflicts involved in making a decision about separation or divorce involve several interrelated factors which are discussed below.

Unconflicted Inertia: To the extent that a person does not anticipate any significant loss in separation or divorce, little or no stress is generated and she/he will experience a sense of inertia and not be compelled to make an immediate decision. The danger in the inertia is that the actual problems and their sometimes serious implications are mentally discounted or denied. For example, some persons will procrastinate for so long that they either forfeit certain legal rights that they may have in separation or divorce proceedings, or legal problems that may have been simple earlier become more complicated.

Unconflicted Change to a New Course of Action: In this situation, the person knows that something is wrong in her/his current pattern of behavior within the relationship. Feeling that change to a new course of action presents no serious risks (such as separation or divorce), the person decides to change and makes a major decision. Although serious risks may be involved, the person does not perceive the risks. Unconflicted change can lead to progressive, small incremental decisions and changes. Hence, a person can make a series of incremental changes without ever canvassing or evaluating the full range of available alternatives (Janis and Mann, 1977).

Defensive Avoidance: In defensive avoidance, a person tries to prevent being exposed to any form of communication that might expose the deficiencies in the decisions and actions already taken. One example would be a person who decides to divorce his spouse and avoids contact with his parents, who previously warned him that marriage to his spouse might be a poor match and even end in divorce. If the person hears undesired information, she/he tends to minimize time spent in thinking about the undesired information. Such defensive "screening" of information is necessary if the individual is to avoid major intrapsychic conflict.

Hypervigilance: This term is used by Janis and Mann (1977) to describe a state of vigilance in which a person suffers from serious errors in judgment, cognitive constriction (failing to see or examine all alternatives), and perseveration. Hypervigilant persons tend to make snap judgments and take drastic, quick actions, which are frequently maladaptive.

Vigilance: Janis and Mann (1977) describe vigilance as a more stable situation during which the person experiences only moderate amounts of stress with a moderate to high rate of vacillation. Feeling that a better solution may be found and that there is adequate time to search for and evaluate alternative solutions, the individual employs a pattern of careful search and appraisal. Self-confidence in one's ability to find better solutions and a realistic appraisal of the immediate results of deciding a course of action, balanced against a decision for a future course of action, are component parts of the process of vigilance. In brief, the alternative of making an immediate decision to separate or divorce (seen as a high risk) is balanced, during a state of vigilance, with a view that deciding later to separate or divorce may afford other advantages, as in financial or emotional aspects of the marriage.

DECISION TO SEPARATE/DIVORCE OR NOT

As previously discussed, decision-making is a complex process. The following five-step model is an application of the work of Janis and Mann (1977) and focuses on decision-making stages experienced by persons considering separation and/or divorce.

Appraising the Challenge: New, challenging information (e.g., that one's spouse is having an affair) triggers a temporary crisis and signals the beginning of the decision-making process. Once the individual decides to act, she/he will begin to search for alternatives.

Surveying Alternatives: Once challenged, the person begins to seek new advice and information from knowledgeable sources. For example, having discovered that one's spouse is having an affair, alternatives may include an immediate separation/divorce, testing alternatives with close friends, and conjoint therapy with a therapist. One's energy during this stage is usually devoted to the discovery and selection of plausible alternatives. A person may decide upon a series of alternatives and prioritize them in order of implementation, for example, "We will seek counseling first and if that is not satisfactory, we will have a trial separation; if problems persist, we will divorce." Both parties may agree to this order, and it becomes their decision-making plan.

Weighing Alternatives: During this stage, the pros and cons of each alternative are carefully assessed in order to determine the best possible course of action. The hallmark of this stage is vacillation. Although the individual may know that a separation or divorce is the best decision, she/he will continue to vacillate as additional information becomes available from friends, relatives, therapists, lawyers, etc. The concern is to make the best possible decision in light of all the alternatives. The person tends to remain at this stage until completely ready to make a commitment to one alternative and carry it out.

Deliberating About Commitment: Once the individual completes an assessment of all the alternatives, she/he makes a commitment to one of them and prepares to act upon the decision. If the decision is for separation or divorce, concern over possible disapproval by friends and relatives occurs. This new level of concern over potential disapproval acts for some as a deterrent to taking immediate action. The individual recognizes that once the decision becomes known she/he will be held to it, and it will be difficult to reverse the decision. The hallmark of this stage is slow, partial commitment over a period of weeks or months. Often the decision is initially shared with persons from whom approval and support are expected. Only later is it shared with those from whom disapproval is anticipated. It is for this reason that many persons separating or divorcing will inform parents and close relatives last rather than first. Once this commitment stage is reached, some persons will carry out the decision even if they have misgivings during the process, rather than face a perceived loss of social esteem for reneging on the decision.

Adhering to Decisions Despite Negative Feedback: The final stage in personal decision-making initially can be a time of contentment, if not euphoria. There is often a feeling of relief in having made a decision and making it known publicly. Having made a decision and acted upon it results in a time of tension-reduction for most persons. Nevertheless, upon receiving any negative feedback or challenges to the wisdom of one's decision, this final stage can shift quickly and the person returns to stage one. Challenges to the newly made decision, however, usually trigger a series of reappraisals, rather than a totally new appraisal as in stage one. Post-decisional conflict is common and should be anticipated in such major decisions as separation and divorce. An important variable to be monitored by clinicians is the capacity of the individual to cope with negative feedback received about the recent decision (s) (Janis and Mann, 1977).

It is important to note that although decision-making processes generally appear to move from stage one to stage five, reversion to a prior stage may occur not only once but several times in the normal sequence of decision-making. A reversion to stage two (surveying alternatives) may occur several times from either stage three or four, during the complex process of deciding about a separation or divorce. The decision to separate or divorce is not a simple or an easy one to make. The complexities involved in such a major decision can be great. On the stress scale developed by Holmes and Rahe (1967) , the decision to divorce one's partner is considered the second most stress-producing event an individual can experience. It is not surprising, then, that a decision to divorce can trigger severe mental anguish over an extended period of time.

SOCIOLOGICAL TRANSITION

Crisis: For some, the feelings of crisis and panic are beyond description when the full impact of the decision to divorce hits (Krantzler, 1975; Hunt and Hunt, 1977) . There is an awareness of having to face a great number of unknowns and the feeling of control over all of one's life crumbles. The magnitude of this personal crisis reaction is idiosyncratic to the individual (Weiss, 1975). Some experience relief, joy, and newfound enthusiasm once the decision to divorce is made. Whatever the reaction, the number of unknown factors one encounters can result in a delayed crisis, minor or major as the weeks elapse (Janis and Mann, 1977).

Consolidation: The need for each individual to consolidate her/his own life and life-style becomes apparent after the separation. Personal finances must be reassessed and additional costs of separate maintenance pose new problems. One's social life, once couple-oriented, changes and eventually consolidates into a single life-style. This often includes many social exclusions from the couple-dominated society. For the middle-aged individual who has functioned in a couple-oriented society for many years, it is a major adjustment to find new ways to function socially.

Adaptation: Discovering new ways to adapt to the single life-style is a constant challenge. For the woman without a career or marketable skills, adapting to a single life where one has to support oneself economically is a serious challenge. Ways in which decisions are made and the ways in which one chooses to cope with new realities determine much of one's future. Decisions pertaining to a new career, further education, relating to family and friends, and even how to relate to children and the former spouse involve social arenas of potential success or failure (Weiss, 1975; Janis and Mann, 1977). It is not surprising that individual and social adaptation can be difficult when one experiences guilt over feeling joy and peace in divorcing a spouse in a miserable marriage. Our cultural norms have favored marriage and the family, with little tolerance for other life-style arrangements (Bernard, 1972). Gettleman and Markowitz (1975) noted, however, that "Divorced homes, which are inevitable in our society, can be stable, healthy, and happy. If education focused more on the process of change itself in a fluid and mobile society, it would be more effective in its task of wholesome socialization" (pp. 39-40). They challenge the traditional view that happiness is to be equated with being married and having children. All divorced individuals need to come to terms with these issues as part of a successful adaptation to the single life-style.

RESTABILIZATION AND GROWTH

Identity and Personal Reorganization: The question of "Who am I?" is posed early in the divorce process. The related question, "Who do I want to become?" is of equal importance. As the individual begins to confront the question of her/his identity as a single individual, personal reorganization begins. Reorganization may involve a change in name (for women) as well as changes in financial, educational, social, and career status. Most experiences of reorganization are gradual (Weiss, 1975). New relationships begin to form. Relatives who reacted negatively to the divorce begin to mellow and accept the individual's new reality. New daily routines are established, energy returns, and life stabilizes despite ups and downs (Krantzler, 1975).

Identity and personal reorganization are established as new life goals and priorities are developed. New values may be formed or modified from prior values. Weiss (1975) estimates that a personal recovery time may range from two to four years. Establishment of a clear pattern of life, less frequent mood swings, establishment of a new set of emotional and social support networks, as well as stable employment are all signs of personal reorganization and stability. In addition, some seek psychotherapy for help in clarifying identity issues and facilitating personal growth in a subjective jumble of old and new emotions.

Family Realignment: The realignment of one's familial ties is a major task at the time of divorce. Former ties with in-laws are changed and the relationship with one's family of origin may or may not undergo change, depending upon their acceptance and/or emotional reaction to the divorce. If one marries again soon after the divorce is final, the realignment includes establishing ties to a new set of in-laws (and/or children) as well as further acceptance/rejection dynamics with one's family of origin. If one's new spouse is a divorcee, the combined double-blending can result in a highly complex set of marital, ex-marital, interfamilial and extrafamilial relationships sufficient to cause anyone a few problems, in even the best of times.

Social Role Reconstruction: Dating feels awkward at best and juvenile at least when one begins to reestablish some form of social life with the opposite sex (Weiss, 1975). Feelings of doubt and uncertainty regarding one's attractiveness and acceptability to the opposite sex plague most persons having recently endured the emotional trauma of divorce. Individuals reentering a single social life need and desire self-affirmation, while fearing subtle or direct rejection from a new person. Social role reconstruction can be slow and painful or quick and growth-producing. Some persons redefine themselves with a "new appearance" through hairstyle, new wardrobe, type of leisure and social activity selected, new hobbies, and new ways of relating sexually. Sexual experimentation is common among the divorced and separated (Weiss, 1975; Hunt and Hunt, 1977). Initial dating usually facilitates role reconstruction and identity reformation; for many, later dating is for the purpose of searching for another permanent relationship. For others, avoidance of any permanent relationship may be a lifetime goal; a second marriage has been ruled out for a variety of reasons. Singlehood is becoming one of the intentional life-style choices in American culture (Bernard, 1972).

Vocational Change and Reappraisal: When separation and divorce occur, most male spouses and approximately half of the female spouses are employed. The employed female will usually remain where she is employed if her job provides income adequate for her needs. If her job does not provide adequate income, she will need to reappraise her vocational future. Further training and education may be required. In some instances, she may be able to move to a new job based on her prior experience and improve her income. For the housewife who has not been working outside the home, her single status may force the issue of employment upon her as a new necessity. Further, a job can provide her with a new community of friends and a social network of personal support.

Values: Separation and divorce may bring with them changes in values for the individuals involved. Values concerning marriage and the family may be affected. For some, a new positive value is placed on singlehood and/or cohabitation in lieu of marriage (Weiss, 1975). Some researchers have noted that lifelong singleness may become more common (Glick and Norton, 1973). Alternative life-styles are the intentional choices of an increasing number of persons (Constantine, 1976; Sussman and Cogswell, 1972).

Personal values regarding money, children, sexuality, marital status, the meaning of family and friends, work and/or career, personal growth, and the importance of life goals may also undergo modification. Value continuity versus value change is a key area for clinicians to monitor with clients going through separation or divorce.

POST-DIVORCE ADJUSTMENTS

The areas of post-divorce adjustment range from children to parents, in-laws, economic survival, former spouse relationships, and the search for new relationships. Each of these areas is discussed in more detail below.

Children: If children are involved in the divorce, there are issues of child custody, visiting arrangements, future education, and relationships with additional children if one or both spouses marry a second time into relationships with existing children. "Blended" families have their unique issues; children may have difficulty adjusting to stepparents. The needs and rights of children may be denied initially, but then erupt in family conflict at later times (Brown, 1976; Weiss, 1975).

Parents: A key variable for clinical assessment is the extent to which the client's parents accept or disapprove of the divorce. Feelings of rejection by the ex-spouse, combined with self-rejection, can be further complicated by rejection and disapproval from one's own parents and even one's in-laws. If the former relationships were accepting and supportive ones, then the rejection is even more potent. If the former relationships were nonaccepting, nonsupportive and cool, then the rejection may have less impact on the individual. The type and quality of relationship maintained with parents over the years will most likely dictate whether they accept or reject the divorce of their child. If other siblings in the same family have divorced in prior years, the parental acceptance may be more routine. The rupturing of primary networks of emotional and social support, with accompanying guilt and depression, is a significant area of therapeutic concern (Weiss, 1975; Brown, 1976).

Economic: Mid-life divorce often involves a more complicated economic situation than divorce in earlier years. Generally, more assets are involved. Investments, home(s), business holdings, automobiles, savings and numerous other assets become the necessary target of a plan of division. Some assets may be liquidated by legal action, against one or both spouses' wishes. A home may be sold, for instance, in order to divide all assets according to the plan in an agreement of division. Economic arrangements and decisions can be complicated, expensive, and painful.

Legal: States without a no-fault system of divorce still operate with an adversary system in divorce proceedings. When lawyers expedite the adversary process and the divorce is contested, legal costs increase while both clients become more embittered. Usually both clients lose more economically and emotionally in drawn-out legal battles. Despite its imperfections, the no-fault system of divorce appears to be more humane and less costly for all concerned. However, the legal complications of mid-life divorce can be substantial, depending upon the age of the couple and their accumulated assets. Some couples may desire, therefore, to work out an initial plan of division of assets and other related matters with the aid of their therapist *prior to* talking with any lawyers (Brown, 1976).

It may be useful for the clinician to remind clients that they should not assume that their lawyer shares with them all of the information regarding their case.

A young couple recently separated were warned by their lawyers that they, in no case, should attempt to even speak with one another about anything, for fear of biasing the case. Separately, each client called. The therapist shared that they wanted to talk to one another by phone. After they talked to one another about a variety of matters, reconciliation was effected with the help of the clinician. If each had continued not to call the other, divorce would have resulted, since each interpreted the warning the lawyers imposed as meaning that the other person was hostile, which was not the case.

Clients need support in evaluating their civil rights when dealing with some lawyers. Certainly other lawyers would not project such overcontrol on a client when the conditions do not warrant a communication breakdown and the fostering of false assumptions about one another (Gettleman and Markowitz, 1975). Clinicians and lawyers need to work more closely with one another.

Social: Separation and divorce will alter an individual's pattern of social relationships. Expectations and reactions can vary greatly, and the client will need clinical support and clarification to deal with a range of reactions clearly and adequately. Divorce propels the individual into the world of the "formerly married," a new social subculture (Hunt, 1966; Weiss, 1975). Feelings of loss, helplessness, inadequacy, confusion, depression, elation, freedom, independence, dependence, and risk are variations of emotional experience which may require clinical guidance to sort out. Some divorcees initially escape into a new social whirl (Krantzler, 1975; Brown, 1976).

Former Spouse Relationships: A range of feelings towards the former spouse can include everything from love to hate and back again. The process of feeling emotionally detached from the ex-spouse can take anywhere from two to four years (Weiss, 1975). The individual should not feel an obligation or duty to somehow "get over" old feelings towards the spouse in a brief time. Children, parents, in-laws, finances, alimony and/or child-support and many other realities of life can provide ongoing forms of brief relationship with the former spouse, whether or not this is desired. Post-marital relationships and meetings are commonly plagued by sharp mood swings, which are perplexing to those experiencing them. Yearnings for the other can be mixed with sharp anger and even hatred. Unconscious collusion can provide numerous "reasons" why one partner must contact or see the former partner. Feelings of attachment to the former spouse often continue to some degree until an attachment to a new individual begins (Weiss, 1975). Fighting and bickering may serve to cover the attachment feelings that remain between former spouses. As each spouse achieves a new identity in life, importance of the former spouse gradually diminishes. A certain percent can remain friends for life; some become permanent enemies.

Figure 1 provides a summary of the model for divorce counseling presented above. For each stage of the separation process, it identifies an antecedent condition, client symptoms, and suggested clinical interventions.

FIGURE 1

Divorce Counseling Model

Antecedent Condition	Client Symptom(s)	Clinical Intervention(s)
A. *Relationship Disenchantment*		
1. Growth or change in self or spouse	Sex role changes, Rebellion, Failure of old contracts	Role clarification, Negotiation, Initiation of new contracts
2. Impact of life events	Unexpected illness, injury or death, Change in values	Routine crisis intervention methods
3. Social comparisons	Judgmental spouse	Clarify dependency needs
4. Shift in rewards/costs	New demands, Complaints over emotional/physical costs	Clarify reasons for shift, Monitor perceptual distortion
5. Third party attraction	Jealousy, Lack of support for one spouse's growth	Clarify unmet needs or emergence of new needs, Investigate emotional support system for both partners
6. Withdrawal	Physical/emotional withdrawal, Small, personal changes in habits	Explore meaning of symptoms of withdrawal, Investigate "message" in changes occurring
B. *Decisional Conflict*		
1. Surfacing opposing pulls	Tension of opposing decisions, Hesitation, vacillation, uncertainty	Focus on client's "perception of the magnitude of loss"
2. Ambivalence and double binds	Good/bad feelings, Sense of loss in any decision made	Focus on commonality of mixed affect, Investigate whether double bind is self-imposed
3. Conflict: To decide or not	Vacillation over making a positive/negative decision	Clarify that no decision is a decision
a. Unconflicted inertia	Minimal feeling of stress	Focus on reality and magnitude of issue/ problem
b. Unconflicted change	Minimal feeling of risk in decision-making	Focus on danger of ignoring many alternatives via a series of small, incremental decisions

FIGURE 1 (*continued*)

Antecedent Condition	Client Symptom(s)	Clinical Intervention(s)
c. Defensive avoidance	Ignores new data and avoids persons who may disapprove of one's decisions	Explore avoidance mechanisms and why employed
d. Hypervigilance	Cognitive constriction, Errors in judgment, Perseveration, High anxiety level, High vacillation	Explore risks of rash, impetuous, impulsive types of decisions and the lack of considerations of other alternatives
e. Vigilance	Careful appraisals, Awareness of risks, Confident of finding a good solution, Adaptive choices	Support the feeling of hope, Value careful appraisals, Monitor reality of time-line to deal with issue/problem
C. *Decision: To separate/ divorce or not*	Decisions are complex yet follow patterns	Focus on pattern and complexity
1. Appraising the challenge	Appraises risk level, Assesses challenge of events and information, Challenge induces a sense of setback unless one changes	Focus on exploration of new courses of action viewed as more desirable than prior actions/ decisions
2. Surveying alternatives	Surveys alternatives like separation or divorce or therapy	Facilitate exploration of fresh alternatives and elimination of weak alternatives
3. Weighing alternatives	Detailed search and evaluation of pluses and minuses of most viable alternatives, Each final alternative mentally practiced, Frustration here may cause reversion to stage two to further survey for additional alternatives	Guide client in careful evaluation of pros/cons of all alternatives, Support reversion to stage two (if necessary)
4. Deliberating about commitment	Focus on implementation of newly formed decision, Concern over disapproval by friends or relatives of the new decision	Clarify all action steps, Accept and support client's anticipated disapproval of decision by others, Clarify need for small incremental decisions as way to test out main decision

FIGURE 1 *(continued)*

Antecedent Condition	Client Symptom(s)	Clinical Intervention(s)
5. Adhering despite negative feedback	Feeling of relief or euphoria, Minimal post-decisional conflict, Reversion to a prior stage is not unusual, Post-decisional bolstering, Overreactions to negative feedback	Support for reaching a major decision point, Accept post-decisional conflict (if any), Support client if any reversion occurs, Clarify need to discount minor negative challenges and feedback, Client capacity for negative feedback needs assessment
D. *Sociological Transition*		
1. Crisis	Feeling of panic and crisis, Severe feeling of loss of control over one's life vs. feeling of elation or joy over making a decision for separation/divorce	Accept full range of feelings as normal part of reactive syndrome, Provide support during acute phase of feeling loss of control, Clarify how mood swings and/or ambivalence occur
2. Consolidation	Reassessment of one's life goals, needs, and identity, Shift to single's life-style from couple-oriented life-style	Clarify the need for a period of reassessment and how it can foster positive personal development, Accept/support fear and pain of middle-aged person facing a single's life-style after many years of marriage
3. Adaptation	How and when to make decisions? Issue of economic survival arises related to future career or educational training, How to cope with personal stress reactions?	Clarify basic decision-making processes including careful examination of a range of alternatives, Clients tend to make major decisions with a "tunnel" vision which precludes a serious consideration of various alternatives, Provide practical stress reduction and relaxation alternatives

FIGURE 1 *(continued)*

Antecedent Condition	Client Symptom(s)	Clinical Intervention(s)
E. *Restabilization and Growth*		
1. Identity and personal reorganization	Questions regarding "Who am I?" and "Who am I to become?" Issues pertaining to partial/complete life reorganization occur including financial, social, career, family and educational	Provide support during risk of initiating new relationships, Clarify why new life goals and values may be required, Suggest alternatives for person to develop a new support network if needed
2. Family realignment	Ties with one's family of origin may be strained or broken. Similar strains or ruptures may occur with one's former in-laws, Relationships with one's children will be altered	Clarify why divorce can threaten ties with either one's family of origin or with in-laws, Provide support during this time until client can find if family ties are ruptured permanently or only temporarily, Suggest modified expectations of self and children
3. Social role reconstruction	Awkward feeling during initial dating attempts provoke feelings of self-doubt, self-worth and attractiveness, Confusion about to whether to marry again is typical	Clarify why feelings of awkwardness occur and offer support during periods of self-doubt, fear of rejection, social failure, or confusion, Clarify that ambivalence about remarriage is typical
4. Vocational change and reappraisal	Usually the issue of vocation hits females more than males with the need for either initial or advanced training or further education	Suggest value of career testing and assessment centers, Life-planning courses or workshops can be a helpful adjunct to on-going therapy
5. Values	Changes in values regarding marriage, family, sex, alternative life-styles, money, career, or education	Monitoring of value change(s) vs. value continuity (stability) by the clinician can be a key area with which to assess and predict overall adjustment

FIGURE 1 *(continued)*

Antecedent Condition	Client Symptom(s)	Clinical Intervention(s)
F. *Post-Divorce Adjustments*		
1. Children	Anxiety over child custody, visiting arrangements, and agreements about holidays, vacations, and education are areas which generate a range of symptoms	Utilize problem-solving approaches (Haley) and clarify futility of person-attacking urges of angry client, Suggest negotiation and/or compromise techniques as alternatives, Facilitate client's dealing with fear(s) underlying immediate level of anger
2. Parents	Parental disapproval and lack of emotional support are key variables to investigate, Need for parental/family support is great, In mid-life, the disapproval of grown children is another symptom	Clarification of client dependency needs and how to deal with those needs, Explore client's support network and what changes have occurred in it or need to occur, Provide support for acute feelings of loneliness as needed, Confront bonding links to grown children and the depth of extant symbiosis in the attachment despite chronological age
3. Economic	Anxiety, anger, fear over implications of any economic decisions for the duration of separation/divorce proceedings	Explore basis of fear, anxieties, anger/rage related to economic situation
4. Legal	Conflict with one's spouse over all the settlement issues involved in divorce, Mid-life economic assets may add to complications of the process	Assist client(s) in carefully evaluating one's emotional needs vs. the economic costs of meeting most of them in court, Explore whether client is knowingly forfeiting basic civil rights to communicate with the other spouse due to overcontrol of adversary-oriented lawyer(s)

FIGURE 1 *(continued)*

Antecedent Condition	Client Symptom(s)	Clinical Intervention(s)
5. Social	Disruption of basic social relationship pattern(s) including family and friends, Feelings of loss, helplessness, depression, elation, freedom, risk, independence, and dependence	Clarify the vast range of affective mood swings, ambivalence towards former mate, and need for changing expectations of self and other, Confront "escapist" and avoidance mechanisms when they occur
6. Former spouse relationships	Broad range of feelings towards former spouse, post-divorce, is often confusing and anxiety inducing, Fighting with ex-spouse or becoming good friends with ex-spouse can be bewildering and elicit questions/doubts about the correctness of one's decision to divorce, Mid-life divorce may be symptomatic of one mate's developmental needs to individuate and restructure life through a divorce	Clarify why mood swings and ambivalence occur, Explore symptoms such as fighting with former spouse or unconscious collusions to still see each other, Indicate that several years may be needed to fully effect such a major life transition, Support decision to divorce if the individual survival need of one spouse takes priority over the marriage per se, Clarify mid-life needs to restructure life and, at times, to divorce as a sign of individual growth

CLINICAL IMPLICATIONS AND APPLICATIONS

Competent separation and divorce counseling requires careful evaluation of: 1) the individuals involved, 2) the relationship history, 3) the type and extent of extended family and friendship network, and 4) other social supports available to each individual. The need for personal and social support is critical during this time of a major life transition. Early assessment of depression and individual psychopathology in each individual is crucial (Briscoe and Smith, 1973, 1975; Overall, 1971), as well as careful attention to suicidal potential (Lester and Beck, 1976).

The decision to divorce in mid-life is often seen as a choice between two negatives; that is, the marriage is viewed negatively and divorce is viewed negatively. Yet, the pain in marriage is known whereas the pain anticipated in divorce is unknown. Because of the marital/ relationship crisis, clients cannot envision the new growth and life-style potential possible for them beyond divorce. One of the important functions of a clinician is to assist the client in examining the cost of deciding for divorce as well as against it. In this context, it is important for the therapist to be sensitive to her/his counter-transference feelings and attitudes towards the patient. Projection of therapist rescue fantasies, values, attitudes, and behaviors onto the client can be dangerous and injurious to the client's struggle and need to make her/his own decisions (Martin, 1976; Fisher, 1975).

Gettleman and Markowitz (1975) challenge clinicians to dig deep into their values and attitudes towards marriage, divorce, alternative life-sytles, and the complexities of the divorce process. They assert that divorce is not always a failure any more than a marriage is always a success, and they suggest that clinicians investigate their own attitudes towards the preservation of traditional marriage and sex roles for both sexes. They especially recommend that clinicians provide guidance to clients with their identity and role-definition crises, which are part of the divorce process.

The concept of a contract is useful when exploring marital relationships with clients. Sager (1976) suggests that dyadic relationships have hidden contracts which must be brought into the open if the relationship is to be treated properly. The contract consists of what each partner expects to receive from her/his spouse and what each expects to give to the other in exchange. He notes that the contents of a contract usually contain three categories of information: 1) expectations of the marriage; 2) biological or intrapsychic individual needs; and 3) the symptoms produced externally in the relationship by problems from the first two categories. Each of these categories may contain individual material from three levels of awareness: 1) conscious and verbalized; 2) conscious but not verbalized; and 3) beyond individual awareness. Not only are contracts not verbalized, but they can and do change over the course of a relationship. When they are changed and not verbalized, relationship disenchantment can begin and conflict may occur.

The model of the separation and divorce process presented in this chapter has implications for the therapist during separation or divorce counseling. The following are some suggestions for therapists who are working with separated or divorced individuals.

1) Facilitate clients in an examination of all possible contracts they and their "former" partners functioned with during the marriage.

2) Facilitate clients in ascertaining whether all major steps have been considered in problem-solving the practical decisions one has to make regarding where to live, where to work, where more education or training is needed, the care of children if appropriate, and the nature and extent of one's support system.

3) Facilitate clients in making personal decisions with which they can live and grow. (See Figure 2.) Basic decisions regarding where to work and live become highly important to the newly separated or divorced person.

4) Areas for therapist evaluation include:

   (a) assessing where the client is in the separation or divorce process;

   (b) determining whether the client has moved through all stages of the loss and bereavement process;

   (c) diagnosing any intrapsychic pathology which may require further treatment;

   (d) assessing the extent of the client's depression and suicide potential;

   (e) reassessing the client's value system and life goals, and assisting in their revision as necessary;

   (f) assessing and revising client's identity and self-image;

   (g) supporting the client in ventilating strong, even fearful feelings of rage, anger, grief, ambivalence and guilt;

   (h) offering directive therapy regarding matters of finances, children, social contacts, support systems, and sexual relationships.

5) The therapist's attitude toward divorce as a normal, natural process with predictable crises, tasks to be mastered, adjustments to live with, and new goals and opportunities with which to challenge the client is another important dynamic of divorce therapy. The dangers of therapist projection onto the client and unawareness of one's own countertransference may add complications to divorce therapy.

6) Facilitating the client's awareness of her/his part in the separation and/or divorce process may be necessary if the individual is to avoid taking the same dynamics, needs, problems, and issues into a remarriage within the typical two or three year post-divorce period.

7) Granting permission to the client to take time to make decisions rather than making precipitous decisions under stress is an important role for the therapist.

8) Clarifying for the client that decisions can be divided into a series of smaller decisions. Separated and divorced persons tend to "lump" many decisions together rather than seeing decisions separately or in a series of potential decisions.

9) Therapists should be sensitive to the possible need of their clients to work with a therapist of the same sex at some point during therapy.

FIGURE 2

Five Stages in Personal Decision Making and the
Associated Major Concerns with Each Stage

1. Appraising the Challenge	Are the risks serious if I don't change?
2. Surveying Alternatives	Is this (salient) alternative an acceptable means for dealing with the challenge?
	Have I sufficiently surveyed the available alternatives?
3. Weighing Alternatives	Which alternative is best?
	Could the best alternative meet the essential requirements?
4. Deliberating about Commitment	Shall I implement the best alternative and allow others to know?
5. Adhering Despite Negative Feedback	Are the risks serious if I don't change? Are the risks serious if I do change?

From Stages of Decision Making by I. L. Janis and L. Mann, in *Decision Making: A Psychological Analysis of Conflict, Choice, and Commitment,* 1977, p. 172. Copyright 1977 by The Free Press. Reprinted by permission.

CONCLUSION

Jessie Bernard commented in her book *The Future of Marriage* (1972) that marriages in the future will have more options than present marriages do. As the transition from traditional marriage to alternative patterns and life-styles, including separation and divorce, continues, it is important to not only focus on the sociological and environmental forces that contribute to these changes, but to understand the complexities and vicissitudes confronted by the individual(s) involved in the actual process of separation and divorce. Although many of the intrapsychic conflicts and interpersonal problems experienced during separation and divorce are idiosyncratic, it is important to establish a comprehensive view of the total process, commencing with estrangement and concluding with the post-divorce series of adjustments.

In this chapter, a comprehensive model of separation and divorce counseling, integrating various models of divorce with decision-making theory (Janis and Mann, 1977), was presented. The proposed model examines the antecedent conditions of relationship disenchantment, the decisional conflicts to separate and/or divorce, the sociological transition, restabilization and growth, and the post-divorce adjustments experienced by couples considering and/or involved in separation/divorce. Clinical implications for assessment and potential treatment applications derived from the model also are discussed. Hopefully, the proposed model may bring about not only a greater understanding of those events that impinge upon the individual considering or entering separation and divorce, but also contribute to ameliorating the problems and conflicts confronted during the separation/divorce process.

REFERENCES

BERNARD, J.: *The Future of Marriage*. New York: Bantam Books, 1972.

BJORKSTEN, O.: *Reaction to Divorce or Separation*. Unpublished paper, 1974.

BOHANNAN, P. (Ed.): *Divorce and After*. New York: Doubleday, 1970.

BRISCOE, C. W. & SMITH, J. B.: Depression and marital turmoil. *Archives of General Psychiatry*, 1973, 29:811-817.

BRISCOE, C. W. & SMITH, J. B.: Depression in bereavement and divorce. *Archives of General Psychiatry*, 1975, 32:439-443.

BROWN, E. M.: Divorce counseling. In: D. H. L. Olson (Ed.), *Treating Relationships*. Lake Mills, Iowa: Graphic Publishing Co., Inc., 1976.

CONSTANTINE, L. L.: Jealousy: From theory to intervention. In D. H. L. Olson (Ed.), *Treating Relationships*. Lake Mills, Iowa: Graphic Publishing, Co., Inc., 1976.

FISHER, E. O.: Divorce counseling and values. *Journal of Religion and Health*, 1975, 14 (4):265-270.

FREUND, J.: Divorce and grief. *Journal of Family Counseling*, 1974, 2 (2):40-43.

GETTLEMAN, S. & MARKOWITZ, J.: *The Courage to Divorce*. New York: Ballantine Books, 1975.

GLICK, P. C.: A demographer looks at American families. *Journal of Marriage and the Family*, 1975, 37:15-26.

GLICK, P. C. & NORTON, A. J.: Perspectives on the recent upturn in divorce and remarriage. *Demography*, 1973, 10 (3):301-314.

GOODE, W. J.: *After Divorce*. Glencoe, Illinois: Free Press, 1956.

GOULD, R. L.: *Transformations, Growth and Change in Adult Life*. New York: Simon & Schuster, 1978.

HOLMES, T. H. & RAHE, R. H.: The social readjustment rating scale. *Journal of Psychosomatic Research*, 1967, 2:213-218.

HUNT, M.: *The World of the Formerly Married*. New York: McGraw-Hill, 1966.

HUNT, M. & HUNT, B.: *The Divorce Experience*. New York: McGraw-Hill, 1977.

JANIS, I. L. & MANN, L.: *Decision Making: A Psychological Analysis of Conflict, Choice and Commitment*. New York: The Free Press, 1977.

KRANTZLER, M.: *Creative Divorce, a New Opportunity for Personal Growth*. New York: Signet Books, 1975.

LESTER, D. & BECK, A. T.: Early loss as a possible "sensitizer" to later loss in attempted suicides. *Psychological Reports*, 1976, 39:121-122.,

LEVINGER, G.: A social psychological perspective on marital dissolution. *The Journal of Social Issues*, 1976, 32 (1):21-47.

LIDZ, T.: *The Person, His Development Throughout the Life Cycle*. New York: Basic Books, Inc., 1968.

LIEBERMAN, E. J.: The prevention of marital problems. In H. Grunebaum and J. Christ (Eds.), *Contemporary Marriage: Structure, Dynamics and Therapy*. Boston: Little, Brown, & Co., 1976.

MARTIN, P. A.: *A Marital Therapy Manual*. New York: Brunner/Mazel, 1976.

McCALL, G. J. & SIMMONS, J. L.: *Identities and Interactions*. New York: Free Press, 1966.

NEUGARTEN, B.: *Middle Age and Aging*. Chicago: University of Chicago Press, 1968.

NORTON, A. J. & GLICK, P. C.: Marital instability: Past, present, and future. *Journal of Social Issues*, 1976, 32 (1):17.

OVERALL, J. E.: Associations between marital history and the nature of manifest psychopathology. *Journal of Abnormal Psychology*, 1971, 78 (2):213-221.

REED, D. M.: Sexual behavior in the separated, divorced, and widowed. In B. J. Sadock, H. I. Kaplan, and A. M. Freedman (Eds.), *The Sexual Experience*. Baltimore: The Williams & Wilkins Co., 1976.

SAGER, C. J.: *Marriage Contracts and Couple Therapy*. New York: Brunner/Mazel, 1976.

SHEEHY, G.: *Passages*. New York: N. P. Dutton & Co., 1976.

SMART, L. S.: An application of Erikson's theory to the recovery-from-divorce process. *Journal of Divorce*, 1977, 1 (1):67-79.

SUSSMAN, M. B. & COGSWELL, B. E.: The meaning of variant and experimental marriage styles and family forms in the 1970's. *Family Coordinator*, 1972, 21:275-281.

VAILLANT, G. E.: *Adaptation to Life*. Boston: Little, Brown & Co., 1977.

WEISS, R. S.: *Marital Separation*. New York: Basic Books, Inc., 1975.

WISEMAN, R. S.: Crisis theory and the process of divorce. *Social Casework*, 1975, 56 (4): 205-212.

Index

179